# Life After Medicine

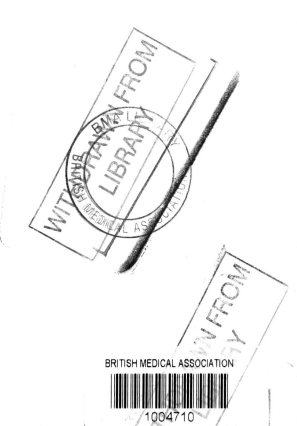

# Life After Medicine

## FOR DOCTORS WHO WANT A TROUBLE-FREE TRANSITION

**SUSAN E KERSLEY**

Life Coach, NLP Master Practitioner and Writer
Retired Medical Practitioner

*Foreword by*

**SONIA HUTTON-TAYLOR**

MBBS FRCS FRCOphth DO
Independent Career Planning Advisor to the Medical Profession
Director, Medical Forum

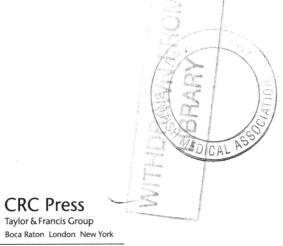

**CRC Press**
Taylor & Francis Group
Boca Raton  London  New York

CRC Press is an imprint of the
Taylor & Francis Group, an **informa** business

**Radcliffe Publishing Ltd**
18 Marcham Road
Abingdon
Oxon OX14 1AA
United Kingdom

www.radcliffe-oxford.com

Electronic catalogue and worldwide online ordering facility.

British Library Cataloguing in Publication Data

A catalogue record for this book is available from the British Library.

ISBN-13: 978 184619 381 1

The paper used for the text pages of this book
is FSC certified. FSC (The Forest Stewardship
Council) is an international network to promote
responsible management of the world's forests.

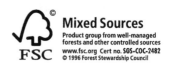

**Mixed Sources**
Product group from well-managed
forests and other controlled sources
www.fsc.org  Cert no. SGS-COC-2482
© 1996 Forest Stewardship Council

Typeset by Pindar NZ, Auckland, New Zealand

# Contents

# Foreword

Given that I have had a 'life after Medicine' for the past 20 years, reading a book about it really took me back in time. All those challenges and emotions relating to moving a career forward into another phase were long forgotten. Yet it was cathartic to revisit them.

My own story is very different to Susan's, but there are many themes within the book that I can identify with. For example, I had only worked in Medicine for six years (compared with 30 years for Susan) before I realised that the pathway I had chosen might not sustain me for a lifetime. Unlike Susan, I did not see my career transition as 'leaving' anything. It was more of a gradual reinvention. Yet there were times when others' views were extremely unhelpful or downright irritating, due to the sort of stigma or labelling that arises when one makes a decision to cease clinical practice. One is made to feel a little as if one has forsaken humanity. Responses like 'What a waste, all those years training', 'Aren't you going to miss it?' and 'Have you been struck off' (to which the answer was no, no and no) were common. In retrospect, the most uninspired and deflating of them all was 'But surely doctors don't need career guidance', given that I then went on to make that very topic my own career within a business. It would have been so reassuring to have read this book back then.

Medics and their families, peers and society have a tendency to think that once a decision to do Medicine has been made, that is 'it' (a bit like taking the cloth). However, there are times when there is a need either to accept that a wrong choice has been made, or to come to terms with the fact that it was the right choice at the time, but that is no longer the case. At other times moving on from clinical practice is simply a logical progression, letting go of one phase of life and moving on to another, such as pursuing some new career challenges.

In addition, shedding the medical career mantle may be just as much of a hurdle for people who are considering early or normal timing of retirement as it is for those who make transitions earlier in their careers. None of these phases in life are goingto be a doddle to navigate, and Susan's book without doubt eases the passage.

So many books or guides have been written about how to get into Medicine or how to get ahead in your medical career – it is both balancing and chastening to have a book that looks at the issues behind the why, how, when and wherefore of moving out of it. This book is mandatory reading for anyone with career misgivings or doubts, or who is in a position (forced or chosen) where it is time for clinical practice to take a back seat after being in the foreground. I am sure that in reading it, some doctors with career doubts will be reassured that their feelings are valid and that this alone will enable them to find creative ways of continuing in clinical work if that is right for them. So, paradoxically, it is a book that can help to restore or maintain some medical careers that might otherwise have hit the rocks. The book raises the question of whether having chosen, for any number of good or not so good reasons, to pursue Medicine as a career, one should continue blindly on whatever happens. The short answer is 'no', but this book provides a framework for evaluating this question for yourself. Those who are nearing or considering retirement will also find Susan's comprehensive perspectives on ceasing clinical practice invaluable in the transition.

**Sonia Hutton-Taylor** MBBS FRCS FRCOphth DO
**Independent Career Planning Advisor to the Medical Profession**
**Director, Medical Forum**
**(an Internet-based resource for career re-evaluation and career guidance)**
*September 2009*

# About the author

**Susan E Kersley** is a retired medical practitioner who changed her life and became a life coach, NLP master practitioner, and writer. She is passionate about enabling doctors to live the life they truly want, in or out of Medicine. She is the author of *Prescription for Change for Doctors Who Want a Life* (2006) and *ABC of Change for Doctors* (2006), both published by Radcliffe Publishing.

Further information can be obtained by visiting her websites (www. thedoctorscoach.co.uk and www.lifeaftermedicine.co.uk).

# Acknowledgements

First, a big thank you to my coaching clients whom I have coached to make decisions about whether to continue their medical work with less stress, or to make a smooth transition into a life after Medicine.

I also wish to thank the doctors who contacted me wondering whether they could enjoy a life after Medicine.

Finally, thanks to my husband and family, who continue to offer me their love and support as I enjoy my life after Medicine.

# CHAPTER 1

# Introduction

Life after Medicine? An oxymoron? I don't think so. I was 54 years old and had had enough of working as a doctor when I decided it was time to leave. Medicine had lost its appeal for me. I'd had enough of busy clinics, demanding and aggressive patients, increasing paperwork, decreasing funding and low morale. There were too many rules and regulations, too many forms to fill in and too much talk of data collection and being 'on target.' Although the feeling had been building up for some time, my epiphany came when I knew it was time to stop moaning and take positive action, which for me meant leaving the medical profession.

Deciding to leave Medicine was the moment when I was able to see clearly and intuitively, understand and find the solution to my personal dilemma. It was a split-second insight when I knew I wanted to change my life by stopping medical work, which I'd been doing for 30 years. I had to find out what else life had to offer. I wanted to do something different, and although I was strongly motivated to leave the profession, I was anxious about all that this would entail, including a loss or change of my personal and public identity. I would no longer be a doctor. Nevertheless, it was the right time for me to take that leap out of my comfort zone into the unknown and find out whether there could be a life after Medicine.

However, although I was anticipating an uncomfortable transition into my new life, I found the journey to be even more challenging than I had expected. Friends, family and colleagues tried their best to dissuade me from embarking on what they and I too perceived as being the enormous step of leaving the profession of which I had been a part for so long. Their negative reactions surprised me and tested my determination, so there were times when it was difficult to remain focused and discover what I wanted to do instead of Medicine.

As a result of the antagonism that I encountered, I experienced several periods of self-doubt about whether they were right and I was wrong and making a big mistake. I now recognise this as part of my journey of change as I experienced a gamut of emotions, on a rollercoaster ride from anticipation and anger to frustration and excitement. In addition, I was genuinely apprehensive about what would happen, and even though I was also very aware of something inside me – a bubbling eagerness about entering a new life stage – I tried to close my ears to those who were trying to persuade me to continue working as a doctor and their suggestions about 'keeping my hand in' and 'doing locums from time to time.'

I had made my decision, and even though I could not understand some colleagues' reactions, I was acutely aware of and upset by their resentment of my departure.

A few people were more encouraging and curious, asking me about my reasons and wondering how and if I would manage to fill my days without the busyness of medical work.

If you, too, are considering leaving the medical profession or are about to retire at the end of a long medical career and are wondering what life will be like, the aim of this book is to enable you to sail through the transition to a new life after Medicine with ease. Your emotions about this shift in your life may be related to whether you are choosing to go voluntarily or whether your imminent departure has been necessary because of ill health, suspension or reaching retirement age. If you are leaving reluctantly, you may be concerned about how you will cope with life beyond the clinics and wards.

Whatever your reason for leaving Medicine, you may be astonished, as I was, to experience a surprisingly strong reaction to your choice, both within yourself and from others.

There is something about being a doctor that makes it difficult and challenging to walk away from the profession, however much you want to do so. There remains the huge issue of your identity as a doctor, not only as you see yourself but also others' expectations of what you can do, especially in emergency situations.

The usual symptoms of dealing with change can be exacerbated by the added nuances of leaving Medicine. Any change may be stressful, particularly if you have ingrained inner beliefs about the consequences of not finishing something, or of giving up sooner than planned. These ideas are connected with how you and those close to you deal with change and regard the medical profession and people who become doctors. Since many people assume that becoming a doctor is a vocation, they find it difficult to cope with the idea of you choosing to move away from your 'calling.'

Your attitudes to life originated to a large extent from your parents, who guided you in the way that they truly thought was best for you. Of course their strategies and rules were based on their own life experiences and what had worked or not worked for them. When you consider how much society has changed since your parents and grandparents were growing up, it's little wonder that their values and hopes about work and life, which were right for them, may no longer be applicable to you now.

When you started at medical school you may have been so highly thought of by your parents and the rest of your family that now, as you consider a life beyond Medicine, you may feel that you are letting them down and being disloyal. However, even though they gave you the grounding that made you the person you are today, you are now entitled to make up your own mind and live in the way you want.

Your desire for change is the match that lights the fire of your transformation and enables a big shift to begin. You may have heard a chance remark, had a conversation with a stranger, watched a programme on television, or read an article, a book or something else that ignited within you a desire for change.

---

Dr Green was fed up with the long hours, and at the end of several days on call always threatened to leave the profession. However, she wasn't able to take the step she needed to write the letter of resignation until she overheard someone visiting a patient, who looked around the ward and said 'Thank goodness I don't work here any more. Look how tired and drawn those doctors are. I'm so glad I gave up Medicine. I wonder why I didn't do it sooner – there is so much else to do.' At that moment Dr Green asked herself 'What's stopping me?' and she realised the answer was herself. As soon as she could get to a computer she wrote her resignation letter.

---

It is *you* who can and must initiate change for yourself. Your epiphany will be the moment when you realise that you have this power. You can be creative about solutions instead of being stuck in the same groove believing there is nothing else you can do. You will find the courage to take action when you tell someone what you will do, maybe by cracking a joke, or perhaps by making it an occasion. Whatever works for you, make the decision and take the first step.

As you begin to talk about what you want, you will find the support that you need to make it happen. You will find someone who says 'I did it. You can, too. You will find life is as interesting and rewarding after Medicine as before. It will be different and you will experience new challenges, but overall it will be satisfying and rewarding.'

---

**Pulsepoints**

- It's up to you to be open and to recognise possibilities when they present themselves to you.

**Prescription**

- What do you want for your life after Medicine?
- What impact will these changes have on the rest of your life?
- Which doors will open and which ones will close?
- What new opportunities will you have?

---

Leaving the medical profession can be a difficult transition to make, whether it is planned or thrust upon you by circumstances. You may experience opposition not only from other people but also from yourself.

You may be aware of an inner voice telling you that what you are doing or about to do is a mistake. Many doctors feel guilty about leaving the profession and worry about how they will fill their days when they are no longer dealing with patients.

Be clear about what you hope to gain from leaving Medicine. It's usually preferable to be clear about what you do want even if your main motivation is to move away from something you don't want.

**Pulsepoints**

Your motivation to leave Medicine may depend on whether you are:
- moving away from a heavy workload
- no longer wanting to be part of the medical profession
- leaving because of external pressures from family
- leaving because of internal pressures, such as illness
- retiring or leaving Medicine because there are many things you want to do instead
- moving away from painful experiences, such as unhelpful colleagues
- moving towards pleasurable experiences, such as new opportunities for travel or work.

**Prescription**

- Keep focused on your goals.
- Be more creative in your thinking.
- Open your mind to many different ways to achieve what you want.

There are nearly always several options available for achieving the same result, and when you involve others to support you, you will have people to whom you can talk and with whom you can share your experiences.

I experienced something similar when I took the plunge in 1997 and decided to leave Medicine. It took me about a year of considering the pros and cons of doing this before I finally wrote a letter of resignation, worked through my three months' notice and then at long last said goodbye to life as a doctor.

I was lucky, I suppose, that it was entirely my choice to leave, so I had the luxury of time on my side.

However, if the reason for you leaving Medicine is something that you haven't had much time to consider, or about which you have no choice – for example, if you have been suspended, or told that you must leave on mental or physical health grounds – the emotional shock and disruption will be very acute and probably more emotionally traumatic than my own experiences. It's not only making the decision to leave that is a huge step, but also the wondering and worrying about what to do next.

My colleagues and even my family did their best to dissuade me from leaving the profession by telling me that I was too young to retire, that I was good at my job, that the patients would ask for me, and that I would pine for the work and not find anything as interesting to do. They pestered me with questions and comments, such as 'What are you going to do with yourself?' and 'You'll be bored when you no longer see patients.'

I asked myself the same thing, and worried that what they said could well be true. What I loved about medical work was connecting with people, listening to their concerns and then by logical processes of deduction, examination and investigations, where indicated, coming to a conclusion about how to advise and treat them. I didn't know for sure what I would do with my time or how I would deal with the gap there would be in my life, and with missing the work itself. I had doubts and moments when I almost did as they suggested and stayed, yet the strong wish to do something different remained. I knew what I had to do.

I was certainly rather hazy about my plans for a life beyond Medicine. I knew that I wanted to be more creative and to do things I had never had time for while I was busy with the demands of a family and medical work. I was very clear that I wanted to do something different – to change my life. It was time to follow my heart and do what I wanted to do. It would be 'me' time. I was confident that I would find something which would be as interesting and satisfying as my years as a doctor had been. At the time, however, I wasn't quite sure what that would be.

I enjoyed reading popular psychology books, and attended counselling and personal development workshops and completed degree courses in psychology and counselling. I was fascinated by exploring the person beyond the illness and finding out what 'makes people tick.' I was sure that if I was alert to opportunities, something suitable would present itself to me – and eventually it did! I read about life coaching in a magazine, and I knew that this was a perfect match for what I was seeking. I decided to train as a life coach. The training involved two years of telephone classes, and during that time I coached many people and also became very comfortable with coaching on the telephone – a very different experience to being face to face with a patient. I also benefited personally from working with a coach, finding time to do those things I was too busy to do while working as a doctor. I've written several books and hope to complete more. I enjoy travelling the world and living by the sea in Cornwall.

As a result of becoming a coach, I found a way of looking at problems as challenges and learned ways of helping people to find their own solutions.

As a doctor I was expected to be 'the expert' and to know all the answers. When I qualified in Medicine back in 1967 there was a very paternalistic attitude to the patient–doctor relationship. Consultations consisted of the patient saying 'Here is my problem, what can you do about it?' As a doctor I was expected to use my skill and experience to decide the source of the problem, determine what had to be investigated and know how to treat the patient's problem.

As a life coach I've learned to use a different approach. I encourage people to find their own answers to their challenges. For example, I help them to free up time to do what they want to do. I encourage them to eliminate 'time wasters', delegate some tasks, do others more efficiently and drop some 'to do's' completely. In this way they can enjoy a more balanced life. They realise that what they dream of doing is within their grasp if they work out the first steps that they need to take. I share my own experiences, if they are relevant, but I no longer assume that my way is the only way. I have become more tolerant of diversity. I am the catalyst which enables people to make the changes they want in their lives. Thirty years as a medical practitioner had given me a special insight into the lifestyle of doctors, so I specialised as a doctor's coach.

---

Several clients talked about their wish to leave Medicine before the usual retirement age. Because I had done this myself, I realised that I had something to offer those doctors to enable them to decide the best way forward.

Unfortunately, because low morale, stress and frustration are common among doctors who are thinking about leaving Medicine sooner rather than later, even though this is a major life transition and involves more than just giving up a job, it is something many doctors consider from time to time. It is a huge change to contemplate, not only in terms of lifestyle but also in terms of role in society and identity as perceived by others. As a result, many doctors go no further than thinking about the possibility before carrying on as before.

However, if you are someone who wants to take that big leap, be aware that when you leave the medical profession, no matter how often you say 'That's it – I'm done with Medicine', you will continue to prick up your ears when you see or hear someone who is discussing their operation or who looks unwell and you wonder what's wrong with them. You can't help mulling over what people say about their doctor and wonder whether you should intervene and suggest another investigation or a different medication. Not only that, but people will still think of you as a doctor and continue to believe that you know everything and anything about health and disease, whatever your past specialty. They say 'once a doctor, always a doctor', and some can't resist asking your opinion about medically related matters about which you may never have known very much. Someone once said to me 'Being a doctor is a bit like Brighton rock – you'll always have "doctor" written right through you.'

If I'd known about coaching while I was working as a doctor, perhaps I wouldn't have left Medicine when I did. Coaching could have helped me to realise how vital it is to look after one's physical and emotional needs, and that balance in all areas of life is paramount. I would have learned about the importance of boundaries, and would have said 'no' more often to demands made of me.

However, I don't have any regrets about my own decision to leave Medicine, and because I coach doctors I still have a strong connection with doctors' lives and lifestyles.

Over the past few years I've learned about and encouraged my clients to get rid of the many things that drain them and their energy, and to increase those activities that increase their energy. This is one of the simple, common-sense strategies which will make a huge difference to your life whether you are in the profession or moving into life after Medicine.

This book aims to motivate you to plan and then enjoy your life after Medicine. It offers you simple ways to do this and so live the life you truly want.

Too many people are living in a way that is not what they want. Instead of wondering what happened to your dreams of life as a doctor and being resigned to the way things have turned out, you can now decide to do what will make a difference to your life.

You may have reached the top of your specialty in the medical profession and be revered by your colleagues as an expert in your field of interest, but if you are not satisfied and happy, there are things you can do to make a difference, in or out of Medicine.

Perhaps you have been on a path dedicated to your medical success which you believed would bring you the rewards you deserved. Maybe you thought that your life, especially your personal life, was 'on hold' until such time, but now, as you consider life after Medicine, you realise that something has been and is missing and you want to do things differently from now onwards, whatever your age. Life has moved on and you are coming to terms with the fact that there will never be that mythical time when everything is 'sorted.'

The most important thing now as you leave Medicine is to stop regretting what might have been and to start to live the life you want without further delay. You can begin to introduce new interests into your days, and when you do that, not only will your life be transformed for the better, but also the people around you will adjust to you, and will change their attitude towards you. You will be different, because you will become more focused, more motivated and more able to move towards what you want.

### Pulsepoints

Think about the stress you have experienced while working as a doctor, and realise that when you leave you will say goodbye to:
- the long hours
- too much responsibility
- a lack of work–life balance
- the need for better personal relationships
- no time in which to do things outside of work.

As you start to experience a life after Medicine, all of these things can be put behind you.

### Prescription

Introduce whatever is most important that has been missing from your life.
- Make a list of what you want to achieve.
- Monitor your progress week by week.

Life is more than just the work you do or did. It's also about your friends and family, your partner, your children and your community. It's about fulfilling your own wishes, too, so you need time to connect with nature, to sit and stare, to walk up mountains, or to be by the ocean. Allow yourself to be creative, take part in sport, play music, paint, or whatever makes your heart sing or connects you with your inner emotional self. You must not forget that your emotions and your body are as much a part of you as your logical mind.

If you are using age as an excuse for not taking on the challenge to do what you really want to do, consider that even if your joints may creak a little, perhaps it's the inflexibility of your mind rather than of your body which is stopping you!

---

**Pulsepoints**

Spend a few hours listening to what you and others say in day-to-day conversation. Notice the words used and the assumptions made. Do you hear yourself saying:

- 'I'm no good at so and so'
- 'I'm dreading tomorrow'
- 'It's an awful journey to get from A to B'
- 'I can't do that – what will they think of me?'

---

**Prescription**

If the above statements sound similar to some things you say regularly, change the words to change your life:

- 'I can do it'
- 'I'm looking forward to tomorrow'
- 'I love travelling from A to B'
- 'I know what I want to do and others admire what I do.'

---

Believe in yourself and what you can achieve even at this new stage of life – your life after Medicine.

---

**Pulsepoints**

The secret of coping with transition and change is simple – look after yourself as well as or even better than you look after others.

---

**Prescription**

If you are overtired and have been stressed and overwhelmed by the demands of a busy medical job for years, take the opportunity when you first leave Medicine to:

- relax
- contemplate your new situation
- decide in an unhurried way how you will occupy yourself.

---

Some people cope with leaving Medicine by immediately becoming involved in too many things.

You may continue to work like Dr Yellow, who did his own locum as well as joining a gym which he goes to each day, taking sailing lessons and travelling all over the country each weekend to visit his children and grandchildren.

What will you do to fill the gap left by not doing your medical work?

Will you take things easy or work a new busy schedule?

As always, it is best to strike a balance. If you do little at first, use the time to plan new activities. However, if you jump straight into a busy new schedule, remember to take a few deep breaths from time to time, to relax and realise that you can take things more easily.

Since your life as a doctor has always been demanding and busy, you will need to take some time to adapt to behaving differently when you leave Medicine, and to change the way you view life. You could compare yourself and your life after Medicine to a battery. Some batteries suddenly go flat and have to be disposed of when they no longer have any power left in them. However, others are rechargeable, so can be made as good as new, ready to work efficiently again.

Think of this as a metaphor for your life. When you think that life has 'gone flat', it is possible to do something to recharge your batteries, too. To achieve this:

➤ let go for a while
➤ stop striving, and just be
➤ remember that whatever is happening is what is right for you now.

| Pulsepoints |
|---|
| Instead of jumping into your new life with little idea of what to do, develop a plan of action. |

| Prescription |
|---|
| • What could you do?<br>• When can you do it?<br>• How will you go about it?<br>• What would you really enjoy?<br>• What creative activities will you start? |

When you know what you want, you can devise ways to achieve it. There is life after Medicine. Find out how to make it the best for you.

# CHAPTER 2

# Not the end of the road

When you leave Medicine you will be doing more than just leaving a profession – you will also be changing your identity and thinking about who you are and your new role in life. As a doctor, a huge part of your identity is that of 'medical practitioner', so when you leave Medicine it takes time, not only for you, but also for others, to see you the person, rather than you the doctor.

You will probably appreciate that some parts of your doctor identity are so ingrained that it's difficult to let them go.

---

Even though I started my life after Medicine several years ago, I still find myself, from time to time, trying to make an 'instant diagnosis' when someone goes by with distinctive signs or symptoms. I no longer want to be involved in conversations about signs and symptoms with friends who still insist in describing them in great detail to me and asking for my opinion 'as a doctor.'

---

If you plan to continue doing medical work even after you've left Medicine, then maybe you won't mind the ongoing recognition of yourself as a doctor, but on the other hand, if you want to move away from all things medical, as I did initially, and to find out who you are without the white coat and the stethoscope and begin to develop yourself in other ways, you will have to be firm about these boundaries and not get drawn into those conversations.

As you start to think about what you will do with yourself and your time in your life after Medicine, it's very likely that you will be attracted to something connected with Medicine.

---

I soon realised that my 30 years of working as a doctor gave me an understanding of medical experience which I could refer to in various ways when I wrote articles and books for doctors about how to have a more balanced life. I also decided to set up my business as a life coach for doctors.

---

You, too, will find the way that is best for you, in which to put your medical knowledge and understanding to good use, if you wish to, in different and interesting ways.

Do you, like many doctors, believe that your medical career has suppressed your creativity? Maybe this is because you have to be meticulous and follow precise procedures, so you tend to use your logical 'left brain' much more than your creative 'right brain.' Life after Medicine offers you the opportunity to explore that creative part of yourself once more.

**Pulsepoints**

Whatever area of creativity touches you, whether it be music, painting, design, ceramics, photography, writing or dance, decide to take action to introduce more creative pursuits into your life from today, even if you haven't yet left Medicine.

**Prescription**

What creative part of you has been suppressed by your medical career? How will you address this in your life after Medicine?

If you are one of the growing number of frustrated doctors who are thinking about taking the leap into a life after Medicine, then you need to decide what to do instead of medical work. Thinking about these things is an important and challenging initial step to take. There will inevitably be a big gap in your life to be filled with something else, when you leave the profession, whether you leave it voluntarily or not. However, if you have a positive mindset you will find something to do which is as fulfilling and as interesting as being a doctor.

When I decided to leave Medicine, what worried me was what I would do instead of medical work. At that time I was convinced my creative side would be satisfied by painting. However, what I actually found gives me the greatest satisfaction is writing both fiction and non-fiction. My experiences of life after Medicine were and are extremely positive and very different from what I had feared.

When you leave behind your very busy life as a doctor you may come to realise how much you have neglected your own needs, especially in the area of hobbies and other interests you had before Medicine took over your life. Leaving Medicine is your chance to pick these up again where you left off.

> **Pulsepoints**
>
> Cast your mind back to a time before Medicine. Picture yourself engrossed in something you enjoyed.

> **Prescription**
>
> What hobbies have you neglected and want to start again?
> Make the commitment to yourself to become involved once more.

When you are considering your options in relation to your life after Medicine, an important issue is whether you are planning to move into another paid occupation, start your own business, have enough savings to make any earnings a bonus rather than a necessity, or be a free spirit without any definite plans, just going along taking each step as it happens.

> **Pulsepoints**
>
> Being a doctor involves much more than the day-to-day work on the wards, in the operating theatres or in the clinics or surgeries. There is also the social aspect of meeting and discussing with colleagues, the intellectual stimulation of working out the likely diagnoses, and the decision making about investigations and treatment.

> **Prescription**
>
> Define what you would most want in your life when you leave Medicine.
> What are you most looking forward to *not* doing any more?

There is also the experience of working in various teams, whether these are the hierarchical teams of doctors from consultant to house officer or the ward teams of doctors working with nurses, radiographers, physiotherapists and phlebotomists.

What I missed most was the one-to-one contact with patients and also the support from and interaction with colleagues. However, I was very relieved to no longer have to deal with the stress of making diagnoses and wondering whether I had decided on the best way forward for the patient.

There seems to be something about being part of the medical profession that makes leaving it easier said than done. When you have been part of the medical community for many years, leaving it can be a difficult and challenging experience, perhaps because of the length of the training and the very confidential and privileged access to patients' high and low moments, from birth to death and everything in between.

It took me about a year to finally decide to leave the profession, and since then I've had no regrets. However, several more years went by until I managed, more or less, to get out of the 'doctor's skin' and become 'me', so I want to reassure you that there is a life after Medicine and although you may not find it straight away, it is the way forward into the rest of your life.

If you are still undecided and wondering whether or not to take the plunge into a 'life after Medicine' to learn and experience things you didn't have time to do during your medical working life, then take time to make up your mind. A life after Medicine is not for every doctor. Some prefer to keep working even well after retirement, until they are literally unable to work any longer. If you, like them, would prefer to remain involved in Medicine rather than take that huge opportunity to explore new options, then before you finally decide, consider carefully what, if anything, you would move to outside of Medicine. For some who are wavering about leaving, there may be a middle way – a way to combine working as a doctor and having more of a life at the same time.

---

**Pulsepoints**

Be aware and be warned that this is a major life transition, and you will experience all or some of the symptoms connected with transition, change and loss because when you are ready to leave Medicine, not only do others begin to see you in a new light, but also you perceive yourself differently.

- Are you really ready to leave and stop working as a doctor?
- Are you convinced that there is a life after working as a doctor for years, and that leaving Medicine is not the end of the road?

---

**Prescription**

In order to get ready to leave the profession, you need to find the confidence and courage to connect with yourself so that you can let the person you really are shine through.

To do this, spend some time focusing on:

- yourself
- your life
- your hopes and dreams
- your challenges
- the solutions that are right for you.

Think about and visualise your dreams, your life purpose, your beliefs and values, your relationships with friends, family and partner, your health and well-being, and your spirituality. When you reflect on your challenges, think too of ways you can live the life you truly want when you are no longer working in the medical profession.

---

You may decide to take a huge leap to transform yourself overnight. However, the truth is that adapting to leaving a profession such as Medicine will take more than a day or two, because it is an ongoing process of adjustment.

It takes time to become accustomed to no longer having a familiar pattern of activities every day. Instead of medical work, you will be deciding on new ways to spend your time and how to keep yourself healthy and happy. There are likely to be times when you experience uncertainty about the transition from your familiar life pattern as a doctor to something different and new.

However, you will begin to recognise a bright and exciting future as you move away from medical work and begin to feel positive about your ability to enjoy life without the routine that you have been following for years.

Your friends and family may be surprised at how you change during this shift in your life. At first they, like you, may doubt whether you will ever get used to not being involved in medical work. Don't worry if this happens – it is part of the process of change, and eventually you will be astonished how you ever found the time to work as a doctor. You will discover the way forward to your new life by being willing to take chances. When you take those first steps along your new path you can judge whether they are in the right direction and adjust them if necessary.

When you leave Medicine you will experience the symptoms of change. Even though being aware that leaving Medicine is a major life transition, the way you react may surprise you. It takes time to adapt to a new lifestyle. You may find that you experience a gamut of emotions similar to grieving as you face the loss of your professional identity, which is probably the biggest change you have to make, regardless of how long you have been part of the medical profession because, like it or not, other people will regard you differently when you are no longer actively engaged in Medicine. Nevertheless, as you discover your new persona you will become aware that you have more freedom to do a whole range of things that were not possible before. These may include starting a new career which may or may not be related to Medicine.

If you believe that you won't notice anything different in your attitude to life you may be in for a shock, because it's likely that your views about what is important will alter, too. Like tectonic plates, the landscape of your life changes when you leave Medicine.

As you think about the course of your life and where it is going, notice how an internal voice speaks to you. For example, if you notice a twinge in your lower chest or an ache in your shoulders, don't dismiss these symptoms but recognise that they may be related to your transition, and ask that part of your body directly (really!) to explain what is going on. Listen to the answer it gives you. It's common to refer to a 'gut reaction' to something, so begin to notice what yours is saying.

**Pulsepoints**

Which part of your body is reacting to you leaving Medicine?

**Prescription**

Ask that part of you what it has to say about your proposed change.

As you prepare for this major transition, to life after Medicine, you may become aware of an underlying frustration which has been there for a long time. Leaving Medicine is a time for you to address any unhappiness in your life and do something to make changes for the better before it is too late. You may reflect now on whether the long hours and the stress that you have experienced over the years was what you really wanted when you started out in Medicine. Yet you may also wonder whether you can cope without it and if you will be able to find enough to do to fill your days. You may be unsure about how you will cope financially, whether you will become a couch potato and if you can be happy without Medicine to keep you occupied. You may also be concerned about your health, if you will suffer as a result of unhealthy habits, and whether it is too late to enjoy better fitness and improved health without becoming fanatical.

You are probably a very conscientious person and, like most doctors, a bit of a perfectionist who likes to be in control of what's going on, so the thought of leaving Medicine may be daunting for you. Medical work gave structure and order to your life. When you leave it you are responsible for creating a new way of managing yourself.

You may have been thinking about and even looking forward to leaving Medicine for years, and have promised yourself all the things you would do at that time, but now perhaps the prospect of actually having that opportunity seems rather scary.

Before you start changing everything it's very important to first acknowledge what you have achieved during your professional medical life, rather than only dwelling on what you would like to have done. You may have been upset when frustrations in relation to work persisted from week to week, month to month, and year to year without much improvement. You may have tried to improve your situation but found that either you lost your motivation or you were too influenced by others telling you that your ideas were untenable. However, you also achieved some positive things as a doctor, so celebrate these now, even though you may have a nagging suspicion that things could have been better and you could have done more to change the system, especially when you looked around at friends who seemed to have got things sorted out so much better than you.

---

**Pulsepoints**

When you leave Medicine you have the chance to build on your past achievements and use your transferable skills to achieve more in a non-medical setting, and to decide how to make up for those things you regretted or that upset you.

---

**Prescription**

Look back at those busy years and ask yourself the following questions:
- What were your greatest achievements?
- What do you most regret?
- What upset you most?

---

You have been far too busy for years and others didn't understand your situation, nor did you understand theirs. Perhaps friends or family accused you of never coming to see them, or maybe your partner was fed up with you coming home late each day and falling asleep in front of the television. You hardly ever had enough energy to go out, and if you managed to see a film or a play you promptly fell asleep. You may have put on weight, too, because you sought comfort in unhealthy food and took hardly any exercise. You were exhausted most of the time and yet you didn't sleep well. When you leave behind the gruelling workload and long hours of your medical life, you really can put all your resolutions about your health and well-being into practice. You can join the gym or swimming pool, take a walk or bike ride every day, eat more healthy food and take time to relax more. If you choose to do so, you can achieve all of these and more.

Whatever your reason for leaving Medicine, something is about to change, and you will change with it. Life after Medicine is not the end of the road because it offers you an amazing opportunity to reinvent yourself, to do things you haven't had time to do for years, to reconnect with friends and family and to get to know your partner again. It will depend on you and your openness to the possibilities that this stage of life offers you now.

You might opt to continue to work as your own locum, whenever your services are needed, or you may choose not to do any medical work at all. There is another way whereby you can continue earning, if you wish, but have the chance to do so in a completely different way. There may be a less stressful job connected in some way with Medicine which would suit you, or you could decide to cut the strings altogether and try something completely new.

Life after Medicine is not only about new opportunities, but also about coming to terms, in a positive and realistic way, with getting older and maybe also dealing with illness and infirmity in either yourself or your close family and friends. Having a positive mindset is important, as always, but particularly as you make a major change to your life you may experience ups and downs, although there can always be something positive to learn even from a negative experience.

If you are very deeply entrenched in your medical role, this is the time to begin to discover who you are beneath the professional facade as you start to move away from the responsibility and characteristics of being a doctor.

---

**Pulsepoints**

Decide that this is the time in your life when you won't delay any longer and you will do whatever you need to do to make your dreams come true, by being willing to take a leap of faith and change the habits of a lifetime in order to have the life you dream of.

---

**Prescription**

Whatever you want to do now, stop justifying why you don't do what you really want, and tell yourself you can do it now because you:
- are not too old
- are fit enough and getting fitter
- are clever enough
- know how or will find out how
- have plenty of time
- are the sort of person who makes a success of whatever you do
- are able to make a difference to your own life and those of others.

**Pulsepoints**

As you begin to explore a life after Medicine, you need to believe that it is not only possible but can also be amazing. Instead of procrastinating, be confident that things will turn out just fine for you.

**Prescription**

To achieve the life you dream of, what do you need to change?
- Change the way you think about yourself.
- Change what you believe about yourself.
- Do what your inner self wants to do.

This book will nudge you, gently, to take the action you know you want to take, but reading and doing nothing is not enough. On its own the book cannot change your life. However, if you follow the suggestions, really think about your own life and take the actions that you need to take, things will be different. Follow the simple suggestions and change the way you think to make a smooth transition into a life after Medicine.

As you speculate about what life after Medicine might mean for you, perhaps with feelings of apprehension as well as excitement about what your next phase of life will bring, you have the chance to choose a different sort of life. You might be energised by this possibility, or you might be dreading the changes that will inevitably occur when the medical work routine no longer dominates your life.

Instead there are opportunities opening up for you, if you are willing to recognise them and if necessary alter your beliefs, so that you can have the life you desire.

Now it's up to you. If you do nothing then nothing will change for you. Or you can follow the suggestions and the world can be your oyster.

# CHAPTER 3

# Stay or leave?

The **advantages of staying in Medicine** are many:
- 'better the devil you know than the devil you don't'
- familiarity with the routine
- having experience and knowledge of the work
- knowing who you have to work with
- knowing where to find help and who to ask when you need something
- opportunities within your specialty
- opportunities to sidestep into a related area of expertise
- the possibility of finding new openings in an unexpected way
- the potential opportunity to combine your clinical expertise with some other possibility that you had not thought of before.

The **disadvantages of staying in Medicine** are:
- the devil you know may be worse than the devil you don't
- familiarity with the routine, which may have become boring, or you may no longer enjoy it
- having experience and knowledge of the work but wanting the stimulus of something new
- your colleagues being unhelpful and difficult to work with, and your desire to work with different people
- although you know where to find help and who to ask when you need something, that help is offered grudgingly

> ➤ opportunities within that specialty, but none that appeal to you
> ➤ opportunities to sidestep into a related area of expertise, but none that you would like to take
> ➤ possibly finding yourself stuck in a rut in the same old day-to-day tedious practice and wonder whether you can ever escape
> ➤ possibly not having come to terms with the routine, or finding it difficult to comply with what is expected
> ➤ your colleagues may be uncommunicative and unhelpful
> ➤ even though you are open to applying for other posts and willing to move to another part of the country if necessary, there may be very few suitable vacancies or you may not be successful in being appointed because the jobs you apply for are very popular.

The **advantages of leaving Medicine** are:
> ➤ the stimulus to learn something different
> ➤ the opportunity to make some changes in your life
> ➤ the opportunity to improve your work–life balance
> ➤ the opportunity to be more creative
> ➤ being able to plan and achieve what you truly want in your life
> ➤ doing what you have dreamed of for years
> ➤ achieving your life's purpose
> ➤ the opportunity to do something completely different if you wish
> ➤ you may have qualifications in a non-medical subject that you wish to pursue further at this time
> ➤ you may want to develop your creative side or travel more. Whatever your dream may be, if you leave there is an opportunity to open previously closed doors to another type of life. You may have an idea which could be realised by starting a business of your own, although you may then need to learn business-related skills such as marketing and networking. However, training for a completely new occupation may be more difficult because of factors such as age or where you live.

The **disadvantages of leaving Medicine** are that:
> ➤ you will need to find other ways to earn a comparable income
> ➤ you enjoy medical work and find it very satisfying
> ➤ you don't want to waste your medical expertise
> ➤ you may not want to learn completely new skills
> ➤ you are happy with the way your life is now

➤ you already use your creativity
➤ you already plan and achieve what you truly want in your life
➤ you are fulfilling your life's purpose
➤ you may be sad about leaving behind all your medical training in order to follow a different path
➤ there may be very strong competition from people who have many more years of experience in your desired new career path than you.

So how can you decide what to do? You could:
➤ talk to people who have done it and listen to their experiences
➤ listen to those who wanted to leave but decided not to
➤ observe your older colleagues, and notice whether they are fit and well or stressed and unwell
➤ notice the emotional impact of the conversations that you have and your reaction to your thoughts about your older colleagues.

Ask yourself the following questions and write down your answers in a note-book. The questions seem quite similar, but you may be surprised at how your answers differ. Answer the questions in relation to the two scenarios – leaving Medicine and not leaving Medicine.
➤ What will happen if I do?
➤ What won't happen if I do?
➤ What will happen if I don't?
➤ What won't happen if I don't?

Which way do you experience the world? Although we are all aware of the things we hear, see and feel, most people experience them in one predomin-ant way. For instance, visual people like to see what might happen, whether in reality, illustrated in a book or magazine, or in their 'mind's eye.' Others are most aware of the world in terms of what they hear, while yet others experi-ence the world via their emotions or through touching and feeling. If you are a mainly auditory person, you may be more strongly influenced by what people say to you about what happened to them or what you hear discussed on the radio or in a lecture. Kinaesthetic people will make decisions based on their 'gut feeling' about their options. They may also like to touch things so, for example, when buying clothes they will want to feel the material before they decide whether to buy.

    There are other factors which may affect your decision to stay or leave.

Maybe you want to move and live in another place, depending on whether you like or dislike your workplace and home. Where would you go if you leave Medicine? Will you move home? Will you travel? Your environment, how you feel about it and how you would change it for the better are important considerations.

Leaving Medicine means doing something different. How do you feel about that? Are you prepared to try something new or would you prefer to continue doing those things that are familiar to you?

As a doctor you have many skills. Do you think you will be able to continue to use these when you leave Medicine? What else will you need to learn in order to survive and be happy after leaving Medicine?

How do you feel about the idea of leaving Medicine? Why do you want to leave or stay? What is it about Medicine which is or is not congruent with the way you want to live? What do you believe would happen if you leave as opposed to if you stay?

How easy will it be for you to shed your doctor identity? Is there anything left of who you were before and who you will be after Medicine? Who are you?

What do you want to achieve during your lifetime? To reach those goals will you need to stay in Medicine or to leave?

Have you ever wondered if a change of government and new policies in relation to healthcare might influence your decision to leave or stay? Opportunities or lack of them in the healthcare service may be related to the political ideas of this or another government. The unknown factor is whether these will be of benefit or disadvantage to doctors.

Have you worked out whether you can survive financially if you leave Medicine? There is no doubt that other career opportunities may not offer such a good salary as Medicine. However, if you have savings or decide to downsize your lifestyle then you may be able to cope well despite a possible drop in earnings.

There may be changes in relation to specialist nurse practitioners doing some of the work that has traditionally been done by doctors, because of a perceived economic benefit of this new arrangement (at least for the government, if not for the patient).

You may be considering a change depending on your idea of a good work–life balance. If this is fine for you now, then so be it, but too many doctors are frustrated by being unable to spend more time with their family and friends, or to pursue their interests and hobbies as they would like to do.

Does your medical work involve you in a lot of travelling and, if so, are you happy about this? Do you want to travel more, or less? Can you get a job in the location where you want it, or do you have to go to the place which is the centre of excellence for your specialty?

How are you coping with the new technology? Does it meet your needs or are you frustrated by how little it is put to good use in healthcare? Does your work lend itself to being done from home, and if so, does that appeal to you? Or do you prefer to be able to go into the ward and the office on site?

Consider carefully all these pros and cons with regard to staying in Medicine or moving on to something else.

# CHAPTER 4

# Six key strategies for a satisfying life after Medicine

If you are feeling concerned and apprehensive about life after Medicine and wondering how to fill your days when you no longer have the routine of regular medical work, make sure you follow the suggestions in this chapter.

Imagine how it would be to let go of anger and resentment you may still feel about the way your medical workload took over your life. Instead of dread and anxiety, frustration and feelings of being overwhelmed, you can look forward to discovering a new world beyond the hospital and surgeries, where you will learn how to have a happy and healthy life after Medicine.

---

**Pulsepoints**

Leaving Medicine is a time to:
- let go and move on
- take your life experiences and look at them through the lens of maturity
- find a new vision, and a new meaning for what life has to offer you now
- have fun and laugh
- revisit long-forgotten hobbies
- bring to the fore those things you always planned to do 'one day.'

What will delight and excite you when you go through the doors to your new life?

---

**Prescription**

There are six essential ways to prepare for a life after Medicine:
- recognise opportunities
- enjoy life
- take time to smell the roses
- imagine what you want
- reinvent yourself
- emerge from your former self.

## STRATEGY 1: RECOGNISE OPPORTUNITIES

Opportunities appear in unexpected ways, if your eyes, ears and heart are open to them. As you leave the medical profession behind, you have the opportunity to do things you never had time to do before. When these opportunities present themselves to you, as they will, be ready to recognise them and take them. Too many people believe that leaving the medical profession is only about closing old doors. It's true that some doors will close, but there are always new and unexpected others which will open instead, for you to explore and consider, with new possibilities which may or may not be connected in some way with Medicine. Keep your eyes, ears and senses alert and you can find amazing ways to have a fulfilling and happy life.

---

Dr Blue became a ship's doctor after he resigned from his GP practice. This gave him an opportunity to travel and see more of the world than he had the chance to do while he was still working as a doctor.

---

Becoming aware of increased opportunities is connected to beliefs which tend to be related to your life experiences, and which can become self-fulfilling prophecies. However, affirmations are a very powerful way to change these and open more doors for you, because when you repeat a phrase several times each day, your subconscious mind 'takes it on board' and believes it to be true. So a positive statement repeated in the first person, present tense, stating what you want to happen as if it is already happening is a most powerful thing. For example, if you feel nervous about something you have to do, and you keep repeating to yourself 'I am confident', you will find that your confidence increases phenomenally.

If you have been saying 'I don't know what I'll do when I leave Medicine', rephrase this as 'I know there are plenty of interesting things that I can do when I leave Medicine,' and you will find that unexpected opportunities arise.

**Pulsepoints**

What negative statements are you repeating to yourself about life after Medicine?

**Prescription**

Turn each negative statement into a positive one. Write these on cards and put them in several prominent places in your home where you can see and read them regularly.

## STRATEGY 2: ENJOY LIFE

You will enjoy life so much more when you have a positive mental outlook. If things don't happen quite the way you might want, look for what you learned from the event. Be a person for whom the glass is half full rather than half empty. If something doesn't work out the way you hoped, decide what you would do differently next time, and take whatever positive things you have learned from the event.

---

Dr Red decided that he would play golf every day once he had left Medicine. However, he soon became bored, as he didn't like playing in the rain, and so decided to move to Spain, where he missed his friends and family too much. Eventually he gave up the idea of being on the golf course all day, returned to the UK and started doing regular GP locums. As a result he was frustrated and remained busy and overworked and continued to talk about what he might do when he gave up his medical work. Finally, he decided to do what he'd wanted to do since he had to give up art in school in order to take sciences. He was accepted to study for a fine art degree in his local university.

---

If you have had to leave Medicine in an unplanned way because of ill health, or if you have been suspended because of or on suspicion of malpractice, you may be feeling very upset and confused about what is happening to you. You may feel angry about how unfairly life has treated you, or guilty about something you did which became much more magnified than you imagined it could be. In these circumstances you may believe that it is impossible to enjoy life again. Amidst all the negative aspects of the situation, and difficult as this might seem to you, just think about what might be the positive outcome of what happened to you, and how you might use your experiences to benefit yourself and to help others.

It's so important to enjoy life, have a laugh, and see the funny side of those situations that upset or frustrate you. Step back, and find someone you know or a group to support you during the difficult times. Others who have been through similar situations can often offer you words of comfort and guidance.

When she was suspended, Dr Purple realised that leaving Medicine gave her the opportunity to enhance her medical communication skills by training as a counsellor so that she could give support and guidance to those going through similar experiences.

---

### Pulsepoints

If you are angry about a particular person, you may be surprised how changing the way you think of him or her can diminish the anger or frustration you feel about what happened. When you make a joke of it, either by telling the story to someone else, or by picturing it in your own mind's eye, you will change the way in which you perceive the circumstances.

### Prescription

- Picture the person as a cartoon character or a clown.
- Imagine them speaking with a squeaky voice or singing everything.

---

If you are leaving Medicine because you have reached the regular retirement age, and you are dreading or apprehensive about what the future might have in store for you, seeing the funny side of life is even more important. There is life after Medicine, but only you can decide what sort of a life it will be.

## STRATEGY 3: TAKE TIME TO SMELL THE ROSES

As a busy doctor you probably didn't very often stop and just allow yourself to be. You will have been used to a very hectic working day, always dealing with tasks to be done, targets and deadlines to be met, and reports to be written, and never even thinking about stopping for a moment or two to smell a flower or listen to a bird singing. That may well have been the last thing you would have thought of doing. However, without the daily demands of a high-powered medical job you can do just that. There are no more pressures to keep going, but instead you will have time to sit down, relax and reflect. You can slow down and realise that there are things going on around you which are beautiful and wonderful. For years you may not have noticed them because you have been too engrossed in the demands of the day-to-day activities connected with medical work. When you leave Medicine you can stop rushing and instead take a deep breath in and out and look around you. Appreciate your surroundings, see the changes that the seasons bring and start to notice the things you used to hurry past. Get up early, watch the sun rise, or make a regular point of seeing the sun set over the sea, look at insects on a flower, smell the perfume of a rose and listen to birds singing.

---

**Pulsepoints**

When you connect with nature in this way:
- your heart will buzz again with the joys of life
- your energy will soar
- you will gain clarity about all the new and exciting things you can now do
- you will find the energy and motivation to start moving towards a new life after Medicine.

---

**Prescription**

Make a commitment to spend some time each day in nature, walking outside, stretching, and doing some regular exercise such as yoga or swimming.

---

Any of these ways of connecting with nature will allow you to re-focus on what is really important for you, and will give your subconscious mind the chance to let you know the best way forward.

Dr Grey took about 6 months to fully 'recover' from the medical life he had led for 20 years. He began to realise how he used to spend most days like a tightly coiled spring, This seemed to relax along with the rest of him as time went by and he began to enjoy his new way of life. He became more aware of the natural world and of his improved health and well-being.

## STRATEGY 4: IMAGINE WHAT YOU WANT

Life will be different when you no longer work in Medicine, but perhaps you are not yet sure how different. Visualisation is a way to facilitate your transition, because by closing your eyes and picturing in your mind's eye what your ideal life would be, you can become clearer about it. Spend some valuable time daydreaming, imagining and picturing what you want for your ideal life after Medicine.

---

**Pulsepoints**

If your life was as you would wish it to be:
- how would you feel when you woke up in the morning?
- what would you see and hear when you looked out of the window?
- how would other people see you behaving?
- what would be different about you, so they would know beyond any doubt that your leaving Medicine had changed your life?

---

**Prescription**

Start by thinking of a place where you love to go, where you can be happy and relaxed. With your eyes closed, imagine yourself there, and notice how good you feel. Notice the sounds, the warmth on your skin, and the colours of nature all around you. When you are in this place, ask yourself what you want for your life when medical work is no longer your priority.

As part of your visualisation, notice:
- how you walk
- what you are wearing
- how you speak.

Bring all of these into your life now.

---

When you adjust one thing, other things begin to happen. Be very specific. Define how you will know that you have achieved what you want. Decide on a timescale for achieving your goals.

When you take the time to do this you can become clearer about how to start changing those parts of your life that you wish to change. If your goals are vague they are less likely to be realised. Perhaps you have already been doing something like this, especially when you are exhausted after a busy night on call or a day with too much to do.

**Pulsepoints**

Say to yourself 'Anything is better than these long stressful hours, so when I no longer have medical commitments, I can spend more time:
- travelling
- swimming
- helping people after earthquakes
- working with children who have been abandoned by their parents
- doing whatever appeals to me.'

**Prescription**

Sit quietly and imagine what it would be like to do these things in your life after Medicine. Obtain really detailed information and bring some part of your dream into your life now.

## STRATEGY 5: REINVENT YOURSELF

When you finally take off the white coat and close the door of the hospital or surgery behind you, become the person you want to be. If you have been a doctor for many years, your identity has been, at least in the eyes of others, very much defined by your medical role. So when you move from Medicine to the rest of your life, you have to deal with both your own and others' reactions to the loss of a major part of your identity. At this time you can carefully consider all of your options about who you can become.

When you leave Medicine, you will notice that you go through a grief reaction because of your loss of identity, work, routine, status and whatever else being a doctor may have meant to you. As a result, you may feel angry, sad and guilty, before you eventually accept and come to terms with the losses. Leaving Medicine is a time to grieve for a while, and then move on to a wonderful opportunity to change yourself radically and do things differently, if you so wish. For some people this will be easier than for others. However, you can expect to experience some or all of the symptoms of grief.

As time goes by and you come to accept being in a different phase of life, you will begin to notice other changes. For instance, if someone asks you at a social event what you do, you will notice your answer and how it gradually changes as you become more used to having left the medical profession. You may start by saying 'I'm a doctor' or 'I used to be a doctor' or 'I'm a retired doctor', until eventually you find that you have progressed to the simple phrase which sums up who you have become, only giving out more about your past if you are asked 'And what did you do before that?'

Decide on your very first step and take the action you need to reinvent yourself. This could be, for example, changing the way you dress, changing your hairstyle or learning something completely new. It may be travelling by bus instead of by car, or finding a different route to the shops. It will also be something deeper, as you change some of your fundamental beliefs about who you are and what you are capable of achieving. You may come to realise that the reason why you didn't do what you really wanted to do years ago was because of your lack of self-belief and lack of self-confidence, so when you leave Medicine you have another opportunity to bring those almost forgotten dreams to fruition.

## STRATEGY 6: EMERGE FROM YOUR FORMER SELF

When you leave Medicine you may experience a metamorphosis. Think of the butterfly and the caterpillar. Imagine that your life up until now has been as a medical caterpillar and now your moment has come to emerge, stretch your wings and become the beautiful creature you were meant to be, living your life in whatever way you want.

Maybe your transformation will be like changing from a tadpole into a frog. That's fine, too. The point I want to make is this – leaving Medicine is a time for change, and this can be as dramatic as what happens to a tadpole or a caterpillar. Your emergent self may seem very different from who you were before you were working as a doctor. However, the seeds for that new creature were already within you. You probably suppressed them for years because there was no way you could follow your authentic dreams while keeping to a busy schedule related to your medical working life. Although you are not changing physically quite as dramatically as the caterpillar or tadpole, you will look different once the stress of the medical work is lifted from your shoulders. However, just like the butterfly and the frog, the imprint for your new self is ready and waiting to emerge.

You can withdraw from the personality you took on in relation to your medical work so that a new one can appear, and there could be a profound change in your beliefs and values, as a result of which you can discover a life after Medicine that is congruent with your new identity.

However, if you recoil at the thought of such a dramatic life change as this, that's OK, too. You may decide to carry on much as you did before, but instead of a full-time medical commitment you might decide to do locums, attend medical committee meetings and go to conferences.

Take a moment to ask yourself whether this is what you really want to be doing, rather than exploring a new way of life after Medicine. It is well known that for some doctors their professional role has become so much a part of them that they find it difficult, at least initially, to identify their true self, which has been hidden for so many years, and prefer to continue doing what feels safe and familiar. That's absolutely fine, of course, so long as you make a positive decision to do that rather than simply wanting to avoid stepping into the unknown.

**Pulsepoints**

Allow the process to happen, and go with the flow, not resisting, doing something different each day and exploring opportunities, and you will discover who you are and what you want.

**Prescription**

If you want to have the benefits of a fulfilling life after Medicine, start to ask yourself the following questions:

- Who am I?
- What do I love to do?
- What am I going to do?

Don't allow leaving Medicine to mean opting out completely from everything. Instead consider it as a time for new experiences. You're older and maybe even a bit wiser, and able to pass on the benefit of your life and medical experience to others, so changing your role within a medical context may be the solution that suits you best.

# CHAPTER 5

# Options and opportunities

While working as a doctor you may have had a problem with your work–life balance. Even after leaving Medicine it is just as important to strike such a balance, because moving from being extremely busy as a doctor to being someone with more time, but with the perception of having very little with which to fill it, can lead some people to regret their decision to leave.

---

Dr Brown worked such long hours that he didn't have any time to be involved in anything apart from Medicine. His social life, which was almost non-existent, revolved entirely around attending conferences and local medical meetings. When he left Medicine he felt as if the bottom had dropped out of his world. He didn't know what to do with himself, and he rapidly became bored and depressed. He sat in front of the television and ate too much. As his weight ballooned he became less and less motivated to do anything. Luckily his wife talked to a former colleague who contacted him to see if he would be willing to do some locum GP sessions. He was delighted to get back into some medical work, but this time he was very clear about what he would do. As he began to feel more like his old self again, he realised how important it is to have a balance, even after leaving Medicine. Encouraged by his family and friends, he joined a local gym and found a new sense of balance between exercise and work which fitted well with an improved situation at home.

---

As a doctor you would have spent long hours dealing with patients and derived much of your self-esteem, identity and satisfaction from your medical work. After you leave Medicine there will be a gap in your life and you may risk either going too far the other way, becoming someone who doesn't get involved in anything any more, or missing medical work so much that you can't let it go and so you continue working almost as much as you did before.

Since you may have neglected your self-care and assigned it to the bottom of the pile while you were working, you may be one of many doctors who, even after they have left the profession, fail to address their own needs with regard to health and well-being. Many doctors forget about their own self-care even though, in or out of Medicine, they have as much right as anyone to enjoy free time away from work, and to refresh and care for themselves – body, mind and spirit. However, whatever your attitude to this was previously, you must address it very urgently when you have left the profession.

### Pulsepoints

Looking after yourself and having a good balance in what you do is a prescription for a better life. The benefits are many, and include:
- improved time management
- less procrastination
- better self-care
- satisfactory personal relationships
- increased energy
- ability to be pro-active
- clarity about boundaries.

### Prescription

Commit to three new ways in which you can improve your body, mind and spirit.

Change something in the way you look after yourself, and other parts of you will benefit, too. For example, when you exercise more you will find that you can think more clearly.

Dr Pink had been a consultant physician who had no social life because she believed that work had to come before everything else. Now about to leave Medicine, she was apprehensive about how she would spend her time without those commitments. She suddenly realised how her working life had taken over everything else and how she had few outside interests or friends. After talking to a life coach she recognised that she couldn't turn the clock back but she could start to have a life from that moment onward. She eventually came to terms with the fact that she couldn't blame herself for what had happened, but that she has the power to change things from now on. She has only one life to live – hers. Her needs and aspirations are different to those of her parents. Even if her father would have been upset by her leaving Medicine, she can explain (even silently) to herself that she understands she may not be doing what he wanted her to do, but from now on she is going to do what she wants. She has had enough of her life being 'on hold' while she achieves so-called success in Medicine. She was then and is now entitled to a life outside of work, whatever stage of her medical career she has reached. She wonders how different her life might have been if she had experienced a reasonable social life.

Don't let regrets about what might have been stop you from doing what you want to do now.

| Pulsepoints |
|---|
| To achieve an improved life balance after you leave Medicine, whether or not you continue to work in medical or non-medical work, you need to:<br>• define clear boundaries, so that you are clear about what you want<br>• delegate appropriately, so that you are doing what you enjoy<br>• be efficient in what you do, so that you don't procrastinate<br>• practise good time management, so that you know what you are going to do<br>• value yourself, so that you make your own life decisions<br>• look after yourself, so that you are as fit and healthy as possible to enjoy the rest of your life. |

| Prescription |
|---|
| Find support and someone to bounce your ideas off, because talking enables you to focus and helps to keep you motivated. |

It's never too late to have more balance in your life. If this seems to be a huge shift from your previous lifestyle, some extra support may be useful. You may have talked to or even have been a mentor during your medical career, so you will appreciate how beneficial it is to have someone to connect with during the time of transition to your life after Medicine, because everyone needs support at some time.

---

Dr White used to love playing the guitar. He longed to do this again, but while working as a doctor he had no time in his busy day, and by the evening he was too tired to practise the instrument. He recognises now that one of the reasons why he had no time was because he used to take a briefcase of work home with him each evening, and by the time that was finished, he was too exhausted to do anything else. He knows that he would have had time to play the guitar if only he hadn't taken work home. He is trying not to blame himself, and is excited about leaving Medicine because he knows that this will give him the opportunity to start playing again. In order to do this he will need to manage his time well so that he can designate time to practise and play. He has already made up his mind to say 'no' to some or all requests to do the occasional locum. He has decided to make a clean break with the past, and he hopes that he can make the transition smoothly. He will need to establish clear and realistic boundaries that define what he will and won't do.

---

Establishing realistic boundaries means defining for yourself what is or is not acceptable for you. This may be in relation to, for example:
➤ what you eat
➤ what you drink
➤ when you exercise
➤ where you exercise
➤ how much time you spend doing something
➤ who you will do something for
➤ how you want to spend your day.

**Pulsepoints**

If your time management could be better and you would like to improve it when you leave Medicine, here are some things you could try:

- Keep a log of how you spend your time over a few days.
- Recognise how you waste time, and then stop wasting so much.
- Delegate what you don't have to do or what you don't want to do.

**Prescription**

- Plan your week so that you do things which you love to do, and don't fill your days with activities you find boring or frustrating.
- Make sure that you use some of your time for creative pursuits such as:
  - ➤ playing music
  - ➤ singing
  - ➤ photography
  - ➤ painting
  - ➤ drawing
  - ➤ writing.
- Being involved in creative activities engages your right brain, in contrast to the logical left side of your brain that you used every day as a doctor.
- Include regular exercise, such as:
  - ➤ walking
  - ➤ swimming
  - ➤ playing sport
  - ➤ going to the gym
  - ➤ dancing.

When you improve the way you manage yourself and your time, you will find that you have more energy, feel happier and are much more efficient.

Dr Orange was a general practitioner. He was even more exhausted than he would normally have been because he had been visiting his dying father each week over a period of several months before his father passed away. He tried to find something positive from this extra burden on his time, and realised that he spent more quality time with his mother to give her the support she needed. He also noticed how nice it was to have a few hours each week to catch up on some reading on the train journey to London and back. It was during this time that he decided he would retire as soon as possible after he had worked his notice. He suddenly realised how much there is to do apart from Medicine, and that it was time to start doing some of these things now while he was still able to do so. He was certain that it was time to change his life.

Become aware of what is missing from your life.

## Pulsepoints

Do you regret:
- how little time you spent with your family
- how you neglected the importance of family relationships and friendships
- not having put aside more time for reading, rest, relaxation and hobbies?

Don't beat yourself up about the past. You did whatever you believed was best. Now you can change things as you enter this new phase of your life.

## Prescription

Take a moment to list what positive learning or messages you can take into your life after Medicine that have come out of your years of working as a doctor. Even the most negative experiences can lead you to a positive message and outcome.

What could you do now to ensure that you have plenty of rest and relaxation?

When you leave the profession you have new opportunities to do things differently, so make sure that you don't feel guilty about wanting to have a fulfilling and happy life after Medicine. Whatever some of your colleagues may tell you, when you leave the medical world there is plenty to do, learn and be involved in. You will have the opportunity to spend time doing what you may have neglected for years.

---

Dr Mauve was a partner in a large practice. Although retired from the partnership, she didn't want to stop working, so she continued doing locum sessions. She was very nervous about stopping altogether because she didn't have any idea what she would do with herself all day. Perhaps as a result of not looking after herself and taking time off when she was ill, she found the work more tiring than she had done previously, but she didn't tell anyone how she felt, and she took self-prescribed antidepressants. She must value herself more and look after her own needs. She did neither by continuing to work instead of taking a break when she felt unwell. She doesn't work very efficiently either, because she may have delayed her own recovery. She has always fervently believed that you have to be tough mentally and physically to be a doctor, so she doesn't want to admit that she can no longer cope with the work. She will probably carry on in this way unhappily for years.

---

Doctors can be very bad at looking after themselves, especially when they are ill or suspect that they may be suffering from a serious illness.

As you consider life after Medicine, take the opportunity of your soon-to-be-changed lifestyle to seek appropriate advice when necessary. If you have a suspected illness, whether physical or mental, you should do what you would have advised your patients – seek professional help. Doctors, in or out of Medicine, are human, too!

### Pulsepoints

You are just as prone to illnesses (both mental and physical) as your patients, and you should avoid self-diagnosis, self-medication, or consulting with colleagues casually.

---

**Prescription**

At this time of transformation don't forget the general principles of looking after your body:

- Eat healthy food.
- Don't smoke.
- Drink alcohol in moderation.
- Take regular exercise.
- Talk to someone who will listen in a non-judgmental way.
- Don't bottle up stress, or self-medicate to cope, but seek appropriate advice and follow the investigations and treatment advised.

# CHAPTER 6

# Seven vital steps

Do you remember back in your medical student days when you used to imagine yourself as a qualified doctor? However long ago it was that you chose to study Medicine, at that time people may have admired your career choice and said 'How wonderful to train to become a doctor – what a vocation!' You believed anything was possible, and you may have thought about how you would be saving the lives of ever grateful patients, as a well-respected member of the profession and the community. Since then, have you ever wondered why life as a doctor didn't quite turn out the way you imagined? Perhaps you were sure you could easily reach the heights of the profession in your favoured specialty, and you hoped for a rather glamorous life, somehow forgetting about the long hours, the endless workload and the encroachment on your family and social life that would result from being a doctor.

Then, after you qualified, you started your house jobs, maybe feeling as if you had learned very little of practical use during your training in relation to working on the wards, and not getting enough sleep for weeks on end as Medicine took over your whole being. Life may have begun to spiral out of your control as you went from one task to the next, pushed along by your seniors, managers and colleagues, filling in forms, learning procedures and being woken up for emergencies.

Over the next few years there were more and more exams to take and research projects in which to be involved, all while working endless hours and feeling completely exhausted for most of the time. You were directed to the next step in your career and told by others what to do, whether to acquire another qualification, or apply for a particular job, without much consultation about what you really wanted for yourself, especially in relation to any life outside of Medicine. It may have seemed that anything apart from Medicine wasn't allowed, so you found yourself living and breathing Medicine most of the 24 hours of the day and night, even dreaming about what had or hadn't happened during the day.

So perhaps life as a doctor hasn't been the pipe dream you once had of a happy and glamorous lifestyle, and you have finally decided that it's time to move on. On the other hand, you might be at the end of a satisfying medical career which has met all of your expectations, and your reason for wanting to leave is that you have reached retirement age and recognise that you can now take the opportunity to fulfil some of your other life's ambitions before it is too late.

---

**Pulsepoints**

Over the years you may have thought about what you could have done instead of Medicine, and now that you are seriously considering leaving Medicine you may have wondered whether:
- it's too late
- you're too old
- others won't approve.

---

**Prescription**

If you have unfulfilled dreams which you think about with regret or longing from time to time, before pushing them out of your mind with a hollow laugh and getting back to your day-to-day routine, think again. It's time to re-assess and re-evaluate what is possible, and with confidence to believe that it isn't too late to change your life.

---

If you have been overwhelmed by having too much to do as a doctor, you might worry that you will never be able to follow your dreams, even though they are still there, lurking in the back of your mind, teasing you, laughing at you, refusing to go away – and all the while you're getting older. This is the time to take a metaphorical step into the unknown and decide on a new direction. Something may have triggered your decision to leave so that after you thought, with a note of regret, 'I always wanted to do that, but somehow or other I never got round to it – I suppose it's too late to change now', you responded 'That's not true – I can still give it a go, if I have the freedom to follow that long forgotten dream.'

Even though the reality of a career in Medicine has taken over your life for many years, you were bogged down with your never-ending day-to-day routines and you have been too tired or busy to even make a start on fulfilling those dreams, the possibility of change is still there. It's up to you to revisit your vision and grab the chances that you still have.

You have spent many years trying to please everyone – everyone except yourself. You may have helped to fulfil other people's dreams, such as your parents' expectations for you, when you became a doctor, and meanwhile lost some or all of your own motivation to find out what you really wanted to do. Leaving Medicine brings you another chance. It's not too late to live the life you wanted years ago, because now is the time to seriously consider the practicalities of life after Medicine. Even after years of long hours, and being overworked, undervalued and over-criticised as a doctor, your time for change has come.

Leaving Medicine means not worrying quite so much about what has to be done by the end of the day. It's a time to relax more, go with the flow of life and do the things you feel most drawn to. It's a time to revisit those long forgotten pleasures of doing what you would really like to do – hobbies such as sport, music or painting. Even spending time with friends and family may have seemed like a rare luxury during the busy medical years, but when you leave Medicine you can organise your days as you wish.

There are seven vital steps that you need to take:

➤ Clarify.
➤ Harmonise.
➤ Affirm.
➤ Negotiate.
➤ Galvanise.
➤ Embody.
➤ Shine.

Follow these steps and your transition will be a smooth one.

## STEP 1: CLARIFY

*Clarify:* make or become clearer

Leaving Medicine gives you an ideal opportunity to re-assess where you are and where you want to be. You can make changes for the better, so you can adapt your dreams to bring the best parts into your life and create what you really want before it's too late.

| Pulsepoints |
| --- |
| Decide what you no longer want or need in your life, including physical and mental clutter. |

| Prescription |
| --- |
| • Throw away the piles of medical journals you thought you might read some time.<br>• Clear out your old clothes, especially those that you haven't worn for years.<br>• Re-assess and get rid of household clutter.<br>• Dispose of whatever you don't want or need. |

If there are too many things in your life which you don't need, you don't have a use for or you don't like – anything from paper to furniture, gifts you never liked to mementoes of your past, medical instruments to pharmaceutical samples long past their use-by dates – get rid of them. Let them go. Eliminate them. List things big and small and then start to get rid of them, day by day.

| Pulsepoints |
| --- |
| Decide how and where you would like to live when you no longer have to be within easy reach of the hospital or practice. If your life has been determined by the demands of others, ruled by their needs rather than yours, and you have become increasingly frustrated by the demands being made of you, moving house is an option you might choose. |

---

**Prescription**

At this time of transition it is important to change your attitude. If you really don't want to do something, then instead of saying or thinking 'I hate doing so and so', you could initially try to make it more fun and you could:

- see how much you could do in the next half hour
- change the expression on your face – do it with a smile rather than a scowl
- change the way your body moves – sit up straighter, make what you have to do into more of a dance
- just say 'No, I'm not going to do that' if the task doesn't have to be done at all, or not necessarily by you.

---

These simple suggestions can transform your day-to-day experience of life.

Clarify what you want for your life after Medicine and decide to make changes, however small they may be. If your situation is not the way you want it at the moment, ask yourself what would make it more acceptable. You will find that when you make small changes, things do improve. Too often people throw up their hands and say 'There's nothing I can do' or 'I'm too fixed in my ways – I can't change now' or 'I don't have any choice – that's just the way it is.' Don't fall into this trap. If you do, your life after Medicine may be as stressed as it was within Medicine. These are just excuses, and excuses can be questioned. For each excuse, ask yourself 'So what?', and then get on with what you want to do.

Look around you and notice which of your former colleagues have already left Medicine and seem to be coping with the issues that challenge you as you enter this new stage of life. Notice what they are doing well and what they seem to be struggling with. Instead of saying 'Well, my experience will not be like theirs', take a moment to go and talk to them and ask 'What advice would you give me about coping with life after Medicine?' Most people will be flattered and will gladly tell you some of the ways in which they dealt with the transition.

Listen, learn, and adapt what they tell you to your own situation. Don't be surprised when they tell you how they found moving on from a medical career into a life after Medicine very challenging at first. Write down your thoughts about what they tell you. The process of writing is a good way for you to clarify what you want as well as what you don't want in your life after Medicine.

Without this process of clarification you will find it more difficult to decide what you want and how to achieve it. It is time to make decisions about your new life and to shape your own destiny. Start to put yourself first. This may itself be a challenge for someone like you who has answered to the needs of others throughout your working life. Remember that your own interests can include how you plan to spend your days, your own health, the well-being of your body, mind and spirit, and your relationships, partner, friends, family and community.

Before you can initiate changes in your life, you need to clarify for yourself the kind of life you want after Medicine, and after considering the big picture for your life bring yourself back to the present and decide what you can initiate now to set the ball rolling to achieve what you want for your future.

---

**Pulsepoints**

From the big picture, think about the steps you need to take to start the process of change, and decide what small change will make a difference to your life, to enhance all parts of your life, from today.

---

**Prescription**

Make a list of the improvements that you want and the first steps you will take to start in relation to:
- work (paid or voluntary)
- your health and well-being
- your relationships
- your friends and family
- the community
- fun and laughter
- spirituality.

---

There may not be an instant result, but drop by drop, bit by bit, small steps will contribute to the big picture, because you have to start with something, however small.

After you have decided what you will do, choose when to do it and write it in your diary to make this commitment to yourself. Then take the action to make it happen. Promise yourself not to delay in making changes, so that you can have more fun in your life now, rather than at some undefined time in the future. For each goal, decide by when you will complete it.

If you say that you would like to do something in the next three months, then work towards achieving this. Be sure that the changes you are thinking about are what you, rather than someone else, want. Is your decision as to whether to stay or go coming from you or is it influenced by what you believe a parent, partner or teacher might say or think of you? Someone long ago may have told you the 'rules' for life, or the rules from their perspective about leaving a profession such as Medicine, especially if you are thinking of leaving before retirement age.

You need to clarify that this decision is right for you now, bearing in mind that your circumstances may have changed since you started Medicine. Perhaps you are no longer single, or you have become single again, or you have a young family, or your children have grown up and moved away, so the way you view life, career and success may have changed over the intervening years. Something that you might not even have considered in the past may be the best way forward for you now.

---

**Pulsepoints**

Become more aware of your life, how it has changed since you were a medical student, and your feelings about making changes. Think about:
- whether the changes you are considering are a 'choice' or a 'should'
- whether you truly want to leave Medicine at this time
- other options, including ways to improve those parts of your life that are causing the most stress, so that you are able to continue within the profession.

---

Until you have clarified your desired outcome for a fulfilling life after Medicine, it will be difficult to know what you need to do to achieve it.

---

**Prescription**

- Make a start by thinking in threes – three things that you want to achieve in the next three months.
- Make these SMART goals:
  - ➤ Specific
  - ➤ Measurable
  - ➤ Achievable
  - ➤ Realistic
  - ➤ Timed.
- Vague goals are difficult to measure. Define something specific so that you will know when you have reached your goal. For example, 'When I'm happier, I'll go to the gym three times a week.'
- For each goal, write down three small steps which will bring you closer to it.
- Decide the date by which you plan to achieve your goals.

---

Becoming really clear about what you want is the most important first step. Clarify your goals and your vision for your life after Medicine and you are on your way to living them.

## STEP 2: HARMONISE

*Harmonise:* bring into or be in harmony

After you have clarified the changes that you want in your life after Medicine and clarified your goals, it is time to harmonise.

Perhaps you have decided that you really want to make some changes, but you are still not sure about your 'big picture.' Maybe you know what you want next week, but you are not yet sure where you want it to lead to eventually. Steven Covey, in his book *The Seven Habits of Highly Effective People*, suggests that we should 'Begin with the end in mind.'

If you want to change your life, you need to develop a clear vision of how life would be if everything was going absolutely perfectly. This means that the more you can harmonise what you do now with what you want for your future, the more likely it is that you will make a smooth transition. Are you prepared to think about and develop the path that you want the rest of your life to take?

Are you ready to take on board the idea that there is a reason and a purpose for everything? If what you have been doing is not what you really want any more, and you have been doing a medical job that you didn't particularly enjoy, but were acquiring the skills necessary to do what you really wanted, then there was a purpose in doing it. In the long term, it is important to harmonise what you do with what you really want, by making some changes in your approach so that you begin to enjoy life much more.

If you take things so seriously that they become a great burden, you will find that by starting to connect with more lightness and tackling things with a smile instead of a frown, you will begin to feel more in harmony with the world.

---

**Pulsepoints**

In order to harmonise, it is helpful to learn and use techniques for becoming fully relaxed, and to practise these for a few minutes every day.

---

**Prescription**

- Take a deep breath in to the count of five, and be aware of any areas of tension in your body.
- As you breathe out, to the count of five, breathe out the tension.
- Continue to breathe in and out slowly, releasing tension as you scan through your body from feet to head.

When you learn to get rid of tension in this way, you can be pushed physically or emotionally back and forth, but you will always come back to your centre of equilibrium.

There may be challenging times in your life after Medicine when you find yourself becoming stressed just as you were while working as a doctor. It helps to adopt this exercise as your stress reliever.

---

**Pulsepoints**

Here are ways first to centre yourself before you develop your vision for your life after Medicine, and secondly to use as a relaxation exercise. It would be helpful if someone reads the visualisation slowly to you, or if you record it yourself so that you can play it back while you are doing the exercise.

---

**Prescription**

*Centring exercise:* Stand with your feet a little apart and your knees slightly bent and breathe into your lower abdomen. This takes you out of your head and into your body and enables you to be more centred and able to deal with situations that might have unbalanced you in the past.

*Relaxation:* Sit quietly and take a few slow breaths in and out. Then close your eyes and, starting with your feet, relax your lower limbs. Working your way through your body, relax your abdomen and your arms. Finally, let your face, jaw and head relax. Your breathing will become slow and shallow. Now imagine yourself walking down a beautiful staircase. With each step, picture yourself becoming more deeply relaxed until you reach the bottom and are fully relaxed. Then picture a door which you open. You enter the place behind the door, where you can live the life you want. Imagine yourself actually living it already. Keeping your eyes closed, take a look around you and listen and become aware of how you feel in your mind's eye. Use all of your five senses and notice your emotions at finding yourself, in your imagination, in this wonderful place.

*(continued)*

**Prescription**

Keep this picture in your memory so that you can recall it when you go back to your present reality. To return to your world as it is now, walk back up the staircase, each step bringing you gradually back to full awareness, take a few deep breaths, and slowly open your eyes. Have a good stretch and you will feel fully alert and relaxed. Take your notebook or journal and write about the place you imagined. Write as much as you can about what you saw, heard, smelled, tasted and felt.

Do these exercises regularly because, when you are centred and relaxed, you will be able to visualise your ideal life, which enters your subconscious mind so that you will be reminded of it as you move towards it.

A good time to do the visualisation exercise is either just before you go to sleep, or when you have just woken up in the morning. As your vision becomes clearer and better defined, you will have a sense of what your desired life after Medicine might be. The more vivid the vision, the more likely you will be to make it real. If the changes that you want seem too big and daunting, you may have done nothing, remaining stuck in a rut and having little or no harmony in your life. You may have felt stressed, as if your energy was draining away, perhaps combined with unhappy relationships and a lack of self-care. These are issues you may need to address before you can make the significant changes that you want. Explore ways to make a start. Don't be like many people whose lack of personal conviction is often based on an unexplored option and saying 'Oh no, that would be impossible – I couldn't do that.' Instead, begin to make informed choices in relation to your life after Medicine.

**Pulsepoints**

What can you do now to begin to harmonise the way your life is now with the way you would like it to be? Define this, and your transition into your life after Medicine will be smoother.

> **Prescription**
>
> - What will your life be like if you don't take some action now?
> - Imagine looking back at your life when you reach the age of 95.
> - What would you regret?
> - How might you complete the sentence 'When I look back at my life I wish I had . . .'?
> - Start with where you are now, and ask yourself the following questions:
>   - How does this compare with where I would like to be?
>   - Am I living in the sort of place I want to live?
>   - Is my home environment the way I want it?
>   - Is my home the sort I love, decorated and furnished the way I really want?
> - Think about yourself living the life you want:
>   - How will your behaviour be different?
>   - If you could be transported into your vision, what would be changed about you?
>   - What would be the expression on your face?
>   - What would be your posture?
>   - How would you move?
>   - What would you talk about?
>   - What would be important to you?
>   - How would other people realise that you were no longer working in Medicine?
> - What would stop you having that life as you leave the profession?
>
> Look at your beliefs about these issues and ask yourself what is the basis for them. Challenge them. Imagine that they aren't true. They may be the way you have always seen the world, but there may be another way to view it. Discuss some of your ideas with others and find out whether they share them or disagree with you. Ask yourself how you would proceed if those obstacles weren't there.

If you do nothing and life goes on in almost the same way, you may have let something or someone prevent you from doing what you really wanted to do.

There is plenty of room in your life to do more than you could possibly imagine when you harmonise your experiences of the past and the present with your expectations for your future life after Medicine. That's the crux of it. First you have to believe that it's possible to change. Then you have to become clear about your vision for the future, by being creative and letting the ideas flow. There is almost nothing, except your own beliefs, preventing you from living the life you truly want when you leave Medicine, and even addressing parts of yourself you may have given up on.

Remember that you will be discovering the 'you' who is different and separate from the 'you' who did the medical job. You may have forgotten about hobbies and activities that you used to do before you became so busy, and you may have talked about how you used to love dancing or yoga or painting or playing the violin. If you would like to do those things again, regain some balance in your life and start to look after yourself much better, then stop talking and start doing. As you begin your life after Medicine, you will find that it is a time to harmonise how you were as a doctor with how you want to be now.

---

**Pulsepoints**

Daydream and think vividly about how it would be if you did all these things you have given up on or put on hold for the time being. With a vivid imagination you can begin to think about how your life could be so much better, if you did some or all of those things again.

---

**Prescription**

Once you have the vision, start behaving 'as if.' For example, if you want more confidence, walk with a confident step. If you want to be happy, put a broad smile on your face. Daydream often to build your mental picture and help yourself to move towards what you want.

---

Change your body language and observe how this changes the way you feel. For example, picture how your body would be if you were sad and depressed. Put your head down, round your shoulders, and look towards the ground. Then change it. Stand up straight, with a big smile on your face, put your shoulders back and stride out confidently.

**Pulsepoints**

Think about your life after Medicine and play with the images in your head, changing the colours, the distance of the image from you, and the quality of the sounds. Notice which you like best, and when you have changed the image for the better, think about this enhanced image at least three times each day.

**Prescription**

Discover three ways in which you can develop your vision for your new life by looking after yourself much more:
- Practise relaxation techniques and use them every day for a few minutes.
- Take regular exercise.
- Carry a small notebook with you in which you can jot down ideas and record your progress.

Remember that what you change now will move you towards your life's purpose – the reason you are here. Don't delay any longer. Start to live. Leaving Medicine can be your chance to change your life for the better.

## STEP 3: AFFIRM

*Affirm:* assert strongly; state as a fact

When you are so sure about what you want for your life after Medicine that you truly believe it, affirm this frequently. For example, say 'When I am . . .' or 'I intend to succeed in . . .', rather than 'Well, I haven't got much of a chance to . . .' or 'I probably won't succeed, so I won't bother trying . . .'

You may wonder why, despite your intentions to do certain things after you leave Medicine, time goes by and even though you may have had a goal for a long time, you don't actually take the necessary action to make it happen.

What you need to do to make the changes you want is to ask yourself what is the pay-off for you of not changing. For example, you may resign from your medical job and then work as a locum for the practice you have just left. You may justify this by saying that you don't want to let the practice down. However, the other side of the coin is that you really don't want to step out of your comfort zone and make some dramatic changes to your life and lifestyle. If you stay with the status quo, or something similar, as much as you can, at least you know what will happen. You know how people in those situations behave. It may seem more satisfactory than wondering how those people might react if you start to do something very different.

What scares you about making changes? Apart from worrying about what you think others would say, you may also be anxious about how you will cope with a new and different lifestyle. Do you believe that others would react badly in response to what you do? Sometimes you may stop yourself doing what you want, or you may continue doing what you don't want to do, because you believe that someone would be upset or offended by your change, as if they have the power to read your mind. You have to affirm for yourself what you want, and understand that you are not responsible for the way others behave towards you.

Other people have choices, just as you do. They may or may not approve of or like what you want to do. However, they can choose how they respond to you. They could be angry or they could be accepting. You are not to blame for their reaction, nor do you have to live a second-rate life after Medicine because you don't want to upset someone.

People get upset, and people can accept that it's part of life that things don't always happen the way we would like them to. Ask yourself what is the worst thing that could happen if the person reacts in the way you fear or worry they may do. Do you truly believe that because someone is upset by your action you would prefer to stay in your unsatisfactory or unhappy situation?

> **Pulsepoints**
>
> Remember that we are each responsible for ourselves. We create our own experiences. It is up to each one of us how we react to a particular set of circumstances. We have a choice as to whether to be angry or sad, happy or indifferent. How do you feel if you look out of the window and see that it's raining? Are you sad because you wanted to do some gardening or happy because you have the opportunity to go to a museum?

> **Prescription**
>
> Notice how you react to a particular situation. Now tell yourself to change to a different emotion. What does that feel like? For example, if you go to a social event which you didn't really want to attend, and you keep moaning that you have got better things to do, tell yourself that you are going to enjoy yourself, how great it is to have the opportunity to meet such interesting people, and so on. Notice how your mindset changes and how you begin to enjoy yourself.

What might stop you making the changes you want? Ask yourself whether these are true reasons or things you can overcome. How is your life now compared with how you would like it to be after Medicine?

It's easy to find excuses for not doing something. If you believe that it's better to keep things as they are because doing something different would upset other people, then you may remain stuck in a rut, unable to let go of being a doctor and thus unable to move on to a fulfilling and happy life after Medicine.

> **Pulsepoints**
>
> Notice where your feeling of apprehension about life after Medicine is coming from.
> - Is it outside or inside you?
> - Are your concerns based on unproven assumptions?
> - Do you tend to think that you know what others would think or say if you did what you want to do?
> - Would this actually stop you doing what you want?

> **Prescription**
>
> Check out these assumptions. Find out whether they are true or whether they are only your thoughts or beliefs about others.

Your hesitation about leaving Medicine may be connected with your years as a doctor when you were too busy and too tired to do much except work and sleep. If you neglected the rest of your life to such a large extent, you may be very nervous about breaking free from the grip of Medicine and becoming an independent person once more, at this stage in your life.

However, you will find that when you start to communicate with friends, family and colleagues and begin to discuss your concerns and ask for whatever help or support you want and need, even if the other person is shocked or says 'Oh no, you can't do that', you will think about why not and ask yourself 'What's the worst thing that could happen if I did so and so?'

The other person may be angry, jealous or sad about the prospect of you leaving, but that is their responsibility, not yours. It's worth taking a risk every now and again and doing something you passionately want to do, which is likely to be a connection with a part of yourself that you have not addressed before. Believe that what you truly want to do is 'in character', whatever others might say, and that it's the rest of the stuff, which bores you and causes your stress levels to rise, which is out of character.

> **Pulsepoints**
>
> Don't let others run or ruin your life. Their aspirations for you may not be congruent with the way you want your life to be. What simple thing could you say to a friend this week which you think might shock them? Go on, have a little practice.

What else might be stopping you doing what you really want to do?

> **Prescription**
>
> Make a list of everything which you believe is stopping you. Then challenge yourself about the things you wrote. Do you know for sure that what you have said is actually true? Who can you ask to clarify the issues? This week start to 'cross off' the obstacles that you have

*(continued)*

> **Prescription** *(continued)*
>
> identified. Challenge yourself to let go of them, or find a way around them or accept them and move onwards the way you want to go. Then you will be ready to move on to the next step.

There may be a number of different reasons why you don't get on with doing what you want to do. When you are thinking about your plans, consider the following in relation to your decision.

➤ Where would you like to be?

➤ What will you be doing?

➤ What skills do you need?

➤ Are your plans congruent with your beliefs and values?

➤ Are they congruent with how you see yourself?

➤ Are they part of your 'big picture'?

As you consider all of these aspects of your decision, take a step forward with each thing you consider so that you are physically in a different place as you consider different aspects of your life. When you recognise what might be stopping you, you will be better able to work out what to do. Perhaps you prefer to remain stuck in a rut, because making changes can be very scary. You may be using delaying tactics as an excuse for not doing things differently. Learn about better ways of communicating so that you can put forward what you want to do without letting the possible reaction of the other person prevent you from doing it.

> **Pulsepoints**
>
> Affirmations – that is, positive statements in the first person which say how you would like the situation to be as if this was already happening – are a useful tool to use.
>
> Create some affirmations that are relevant to your situation. For example:
>
> • I succeed effortlessly in my life after Medicine.
> • I live a life of true happiness after Medicine.
> • I am confident in everything I do during my life after Medicine.

**Prescription**

Create several appropriate affirmations which would be useful for you and which describe how you want your life after Medicine to be. Then make a commitment to repeat them at least 100 times a day so that your subconscious mind begins to believe that they are already happening.

## STEP 4: NEGOTIATE

***Negotiate:*** find a way over or through an obstacle or difficulty; confer with others to reach a compromise or agreement

Being able to negotiate is a skill that you need to develop if you want a life after Medicine.

---

### Pulsepoints

People and situations may seem to be blocking your progress and stopping you. Is your rationale really about you not wanting to change? Is your justification for your lack of progress about you not having the confidence or knowing how to approach another person to ask for something different?

---

### Prescription

- Make a list of who you need to talk to.
- Decide who to confer with, to reach an agreement or a compromise, in order to overcome these difficulties.
- List five excuses for not changing that you are you using. What do you notice about these?
- List at least ten ways to set yourself in the right direction for change.
- Be pro-active.

---

Life after Medicine is an opportunity for new learning, and also gives you the chance to catch up with unfinished business. There may be books that you always wanted to read and, even though you bought them, you never got around to reading. Without the long hours of medical work and the expectation that you will keep up with the latest journal issues, you could indulge yourself by designating some time each day to curl up in your favourite armchair and get lost in a gripping novel, or use the opportunity to learn new skills.

Did you concentrate on science at school in order to study Medicine, yet always wish that you knew more about history or geography? What have you always wanted to learn? Have you wanted to increase your understanding of art or music?

With whom must you negotiate to make a start on your new projects? Sometimes the answer is yourself, because if you can't get going on your first step you can ask yourself all the questions necessary to find out where the block might be. Perhaps your first step is too big. Carry on asking yourself 'What do I have to do before that?', and as you keep repeating that question you will eventually get to the correct first step, however small it may be. Then you can move on to the next step, and the next one. Remember that nothing will change unless you take some action. It has to be you who takes this action. Only you can change – you cannot change other people. However, when you change they will alter their response to you.

Quite often what stops you moving forward is fear of:

➤ what might happen when you change
➤ how others might respond differently to you
➤ giving up a well-established lifestyle
➤ going into the unknown.

Since your life after Medicine is likely to involve other people, you need to negotiate with them.

A good way to do this, especially if you have something to say which you think the other person may not approve of, is to use a 'positive sandwich.' The next time you have to ask for something which you find awkward or unpleasant for yourself or for the other person, try this technique. Before you start, make sure that you have established a rapport with the other person by matching and mirroring their body language, their tone of voice and their rate of breathing.

Start with the white fluffy stuff. Tell them how much you've learned or how much you appreciate what they do, or something else flattering. Then follow this with the meat of what you want to say. Finally, close with some more complimentary remarks – more fluffy stuff. Make sure that you explain your situation and then make a request – tell them what you want from them and by when. Don't expect them to be able to read your mind. Once you have made the request, wait to hear whether what you asked for has been heard. Then note whether the other person has agreed to do what you asked of them. Don't assume that just asking for something means automatic fulfilment.

Sometimes assumptions are made about what the other person will or won't do because they haven't actually agreed to do anything, or you didn't explain specifically what you wanted.

You may approach a friend and say 'I want to do things differently when I leave Medicine, but I may not be able to cope with this change in my life on my own – I need some support', and you may not get what you actually need. However, if instead you say 'I'm finding the transition from Medicine quite challenging. I know you've come through a similar change very successfully. What I need is someone like you who understands what I'm going through. Could we meet about once a week, for the next month or two and talk about what's going on for me?', you are more likely to obtain an appropriate response. If the other person says 'no' to your request, you may have to negotiate with them or find someone else. If they aren't prepared to do what you want, ask them what they are able to offer you in the way of support.

Another doctor may express his apprehension like this:

> I'll be doing things differently when I don't go to the practice any more, and I know that goes along with the way my life will change. Even though it's my decision to leave Medicine and I'm looking forward to having more chance to do other things, I'm feeling a bit anxious about coping without the routine of medical work. As you've been through this transition yourself a few years ago, I'd really appreciate some support from you as I discover new ways to organise my days. By support what I mean is this – I'd like to have the opportunity to talk to you about once a week for the next few weeks. I really just want you to listen, not criticise, but be there for me to bounce some ideas off. However, if you can offer some constructive comments without being affected by whether or not I do what you suggest, I would be very grateful. Could you do that for me?

The answer might be:

> I'd be happy to do that. However, I can only meet you about once a month, because since I left Medicine I've become very busy with various projects. However, if you ever want to pick up the phone and chat, I'll be happy to give you that support. If you are anything like me, you'll find your new feet very quickly. Your medical background will have prepared you to be very organised and motivated.

## STEP 5: GALVANISE

*Galvanise:* rouse forcefully, especially by shock or by excitement; stimulate as if by electricity; thrill, energise, inspire into action

However wonderful your plans and intentions for a life after Medicine may be, nothing much will change unless you take action. Remember that some people even make quite definite decisions, yet don't do anything. That first step out of your comfort zone sometimes seems far too daunting to take. However, be assured that when you find the courage to do so, it mostly turns out to be much easier than you had been dreading! What you need to do is to galvanise yourself into taking that action, by using the passion that comes from within yourself. When you are excited and feel very strongly about what you are going to do in your life after Medicine, you will find the courage and strength to cross that line – so much so that when you do cross it, you will be an inspiration to others who want to do the same. If you aren't passionate about what you want, think again, as you may not have set the goals which are right for you, in which case you will lack motivation.

When you are ready to galvanise yourself to put your plans into action and move on to the next stage, you will be able take the appropriate action to get started. Remember that you can plan and plan, but ultimately nothing changes until you do something differently.

---

### Pulsepoints

What will be your first step in the direction that you want to go? It could be something very small, such as:

- making a few phone calls
- writing a letter
- arranging to meet someone who might give you an insight into the opportunities and challenges of life after Medicine.

Listen and discuss, but in the end the passion has to be yours, based on what you have learned and your expectations. Others may not understand why you want to leave Medicine, and that is fine, because you are the one making the decision to do that, not them. Listen to what they tell you, weigh up the pros and cons and then make the decision for yourself according to your needs, beliefs, feelings and wishes. But be wary, and remember that the other person may have a very different life experience.

---

**Prescription**

To decide which choice is best for you, imagine that you could hold option 1 and option 2 in each hand. Notice whether one feels heavier than the other. Then let options 1 and 2 talk to each other and justify why they are the choice you must make. Look at one hand as you do this and ask it to tell you the reasons why you should choose it. Say out loud the words that choice would tell you. Then look at the other hand and ask it to tell you the reasons for choosing it. Allow the options to have a conversation with each other until they have said all that they want to say. Then, thinking about the positive points for each option, bring your hands together and ask whether there is a way to integrate the best reasons from both and how you might be able to do this. This may bring up a third option that you hadn't considered before, or you may realise that you could adapt one of the options to incorporate the best parts of the other option, taking the integrated idea and considering what to do next.

---

Moving forward and taking action is the next step when you have thought about what you could do to have the life you dream of after Medicine. Make an action plan by writing down the various stages you will need to complete before you can get to where you want to go. For example, if you would love to do a part-time course but have no idea where you can do it, when the next course starts, how much it will cost, or when you have to apply for it, then you will remain stuck in your inactivity. Find out some facts. Is what you want to do possible? You must find out the practical information before you can make an informed decision. It's too easy to dismiss what you want to do by saying 'I'd be too old to apply for that' or 'I wouldn't have the time.'

When you have the facts, you will have a basis for deciding whether your idea is feasible or not. If you really want something, don't give up at the first hurdle, but work out ways to overcome the challenges.

---

**Pulsepoints**

Stop making assumptions. If you really want something to happen in your life after Medicine that isn't in your life right now, it's important to look at how to achieve it.

> **Prescription**
>
> Don't limit yourself. Instead, consider:
> - being more open to other possibilities
> - finding out how much they will cost
> - quantifying the value of living a life you love
> - measuring value in relation to money paid out
> - who you know who could help
> - who in your network could support and encourage you.

Beware of people, who may be quite close to you, who have their own agenda and who don't want you to change because it will upset their lives.

It can be useful to talk to someone from outside your own life who can be objective when you talk things through with them. A coach is someone off whom you can bounce your ideas. They can help you to see other possible solutions to a dilemma.

---

Dr Black didn't want to give up Medicine altogether when he retired, but he no longer wanted the commitment and stress of general practice. He loved travelling, and was attracted to the idea of becoming a ship's doctor. This turned out to be an ideal solution. He worked on cruise ships a couple of times a year, and enjoyed free passage for himself and his wife while they visited many parts of the world they had wanted to see in return for a few hours' work each day with passengers who sought medical advice from him.

---

Galvanise yourself to find the way forward for yourself and begin to have a great, rewarding life after Medicine.

## STEP 6: EMBODY

***Embody:*** give concrete or discernible form to an idea; be an expression of an idea; form into a body

In order to live the life you want after leaving Medicine and make the changes necessary to create it, you need to embody them. One way to do this is by repeating affirmations regularly so that you give your subconscious mind the important messages. As mentioned earlier, when you keep repeating a statement that begins 'I am . . .' as if what you want is already present in your life, your subconscious mind will eventually allow transformation to happen.

In order to know what to affirm, you have to get into the body, so to speak, of someone who is already living the kind of life you want. The way to do this is to picture yourself already experiencing such a life. Perhaps you could imagine the situation as if you are watching a film on a cinema screen. As you watch yourself, make the picture brighter, make the sounds clearer and connect with your emotions. Then imagine yourself stepping into the film and into the character whom you have been watching on the screen.

How does the new you walk and talk? Notice these things, and then start to bring them into your present life.

---

When I worked as a doctor, most female medics wore skirts rather than trousers. From the day I handed in my letter of resignation until I left three months later I never wore a skirt to work again! I soon got used to wearing trousers every day. At the time it seemed quite a daring thing to do, and it certainly helped me to show the world I was about to be making more changes to my lifestyle.

---

If you walk the way someone who has achieved what you hope to achieve would walk, you will appear more self-confident and, surprisingly, you will find that you can deal with difficult situations more easily.

---

I certainly found a new confidence knowing I was going to leave, and I became more assertive and found it easier to say 'no.'

---

What can you do if you don't really know what you want but only that you've had enough of things as they are now? You are still looking for answers, even though you are now sure of the question. Although moving away from something you don't like is a strong incentive for so doing, you will find that your driving force will be much more powerful and long-lasting if you define what it is you are moving towards.

Although I wasn't completely clear about what I wanted when I left Medicine, I was clear about wanting to be more creative, and doing something which involved interacting with other people in a caring and helping capacity. I was very aware that these desires were embodied within me and were congruent with my values. They gelled perfectly and satisfied what I wanted for my life after Medicine when I discovered coaching and writing.

Perhaps in the past you might have carried on with a resigned shrug and a 'Well, this is what life is about, isn't it?' kind of expression. Now at last you recognise that things could be different and that you are not prepared to continue in the same way for the rest of your life.

Even though she had accepted being retired, Dr Silver found it difficult to let go of thinking of herself as a doctor. During many years as a doctor she had embodied the word 'doctor', as do most doctors. She continued to say 'I'm a doctor' for several years, until she was ready to let that go and begin to get into her new self for her life after Medicine.

You may feel that you want some new ideas. However, it is very probable that all the ideas you could possibly want or need are already within you. You have to recognise them for what they are and have the courage to look at them, hear what they are saying to you and bring them out into the open so that they can develop. When you do this, you may find that some of them are in quite embryonic form, and you will need to explore them further with someone who has done something similar. How can you access your internal wealth of ideas? How can you embody them?

Create some space, both emotional and physical, for these new hopes and dreams to pour into. Take time to sit quietly, or go for a walk on your own in the countryside, by the sea, or to a peaceful place where you can allow your imagination to flow. Don't talk. Some people find that listening to music or meditating helps them to discover new ideas. Just allow whatever is in your subconscious mind to come into your conscious mind. As you begin this exercise, ask yourself what you want to find out and what resources you most need. Keep your notebook and a pen with you so that you can jot down your thoughts.

When you walk, your steps become part of the rhythm of your life. Walking has been referred to by Julia Cameron as a moving meditation, because all sorts of ideas may pop into your mind. Either write them down then and there, or dictate them into a small audio recorder. If you don't do so, you may wonder later what it was you were so excited about.

Similarly, other forms of exercise such as swimming or free-form dancing may enable thoughts and ideas to appear. Regular aerobic exercise also helps you to become fitter, and the release of endorphins makes you feel good.

Maybe you need to have a bit of a 'clear out,' both mentally and physically, to prepare yourself for your life after Medicine. They say that nature abhors a vacuum, and so it seems to be. When you start to clear away a lot of physical clutter, or put emotional clutter into your 'mental shredder', there seems to be more space available into which new ideas and opportunities can come.

Make a list of everything that gets on your nerves – at least five things, but preferably about 50. Start with the easy things, and eliminate them one by one. It's a great feeling when you can cross each item off your long 'to do' list. Get them done, or ask someone else to do them – for payment, or as a favour, or as an exchange.

Stop putting things off. Just do them as you realise they need doing. Decide how long the task will take to do, designate a time for it, and write the task in your diary with that amount of time blocked off. If the task might take 3 hours and you only have 15-minute slots, divide the big task into smaller ones. That way you will make progress.

Decide what action you will take this week in order to embody bit by bit, step by step, the new you – who lives the life you want to live. What will you decide to do before you can move on to the next step? When will you take the steps that you need to take? Make a list of the things you are going to do, make your mind up and then do them. Embody the changes that you want.

## STEP 7: SHINE

*Shine:* emit or reflect light; be bright; glow; be visible; not be obscured by clouds; excel; be brilliant: look healthy; radiate; be expert; be outstanding; be a star

It is satisfying to do something special, just for you, as a celebration of what you have accomplished in order to reach this stage of your life. It is good to recognise what you have done for your patients. As you move into a life after Medicine, recognise, too, that there is so much more you can do and achieve from now on. It is great to reward yourself for all the things you have been successful in and the way all those life experiences will be important in whatever you choose to do now. Your life as a doctor will have inspired others, and you may want to keep a 'finger on the pulse' by becoming a mentor to younger doctors and so passing on to them the benefit of your knowledge and skills.

As you explore the way your life will change when you leave Medicine, remember to congratulate yourself as you learn new skills and deal with your challenges effectively. Looking forward to a special treat can be an incentive to get something done.

Notice what happens to your physiology when you shine. Become aware of how your body language, your mood and your expression change when you feel pleased with yourself. Realise that you are an inspiration to others and celebrate.

Treat yourself. How can you do that? Note five ways to offer yourself a gift or a treat for the things you have achieved in your life up until now, and for what you have done in the past few weeks and days since you decided things have to change for the better.

Here are some ideas. You could go for a walk in nature, relax in a spa, have a massage, go out to a restaurant with someone special, see a good film, or even allow yourself the luxury of just sitting and thinking. Doing something out of the ordinary for yourself is very important for raising your self-esteem, valuing yourself and acknowledging that you deserve something, too. It's easy to be always doing things for other people and to forget about your own needs. If you are someone who is waiting for your nearest and dearest to accept what it is you need to feel good about yourself, then perhaps now is the time to ask for what you want. Are you ready for the challenge? Make a list of what makes you shine even more. What gives you a buzz? Make a pledge to do some of these things this week. Make a commitment to yourself to look after yourself much, much better.

The synchronicity of the universe means that everything is interconnected.

Whatever changes you initiate will make other things and other people change, too. You will be different, and when you shine you will motivate others, be outstanding, happy and healthy, and so will those around you when they feel your radiance. You can live a life in which you are contented and fulfilled.

However, for the seven vital steps to transform your life, you have to do more than just read about them. You must make a promise to yourself to put some or all of what you have read into practice. When you fully engage in the process of change your view of the world will alter, things you thought were impossible to do while you were a busy doctor will become achievable, and you will wonder why you procrastinated for so long. It is just like a spreadsheet – when you change one thing, everything else changes as well.

# CHAPTER 7

# Reflections on life after Medicine and retirement

You may be one of those doctors who doesn't want to give up all things medical completely because Medicine has been so much a part of your life for so long, and the very nature of the job means that it is difficult for a doctor, at the end of the working day or night, to go home and forget about all the things they have seen and experienced. It is certainly not compulsory to sever all links with Medicine and the medical profession when you decide to leave it.

Medicine is so much more than a routine job because you are dealing with people and all those indefinable factors that contribute to every doctor–patient interaction, other than just the history taking, examination, investigation and treatment. There is also the way you communicate, how you react to each other's appearance and the hidden agendas you both have – for example, what the patient fears, and how you react to their comments. You don't forget the times when you were very tired and responded angrily to a patient's demands, which may in fact have been quite reasonable, nor do you forget the delightful people who had terrible diagnoses and prognoses. You took these and many other worries and stresses home with you and maybe found a sympathetic person to talk to, or maybe not. Being a doctor permeates your entire being. It is who and what you are for many years. The idea of a life beyond Medicine may seem impossible, even to those who make a positive choice to leave and are already clear about what they will do. They may wonder if they will ever be able to fill the void left by such a major part of their life not being there any more.

Since a common reason for leaving Medicine is that you no longer want to work such long hours and would prefer something more fluid instead, you may look for and discover something else to do which is different, but which has some link to Medicine.

---

That can happen even if initially, like me, you don't want to do anything medical. Despite feeling like this, I found that there was something which drew me back into the medical world, even if somewhat on the periphery, as a life coach for doctors, and for me that was the connection I wanted – something completely different and yet somehow associated.

---

You really can have a life after Medicine, and as you begin to explore the possibilities you will become more confident that the best is yet to come. You will be able to pass on the benefits of your life and medical experiences to others, too. But that is not all. You can enjoy whatever this phase of your life has to offer you in the way of new learning, and you can begin to fulfil your life's purpose. If part of your life's purpose has been to treat patients, this can continue when you leave Medicine – for example, if you are a mentor to other doctors or a medical adviser to organisations or the media.

---

Dr Gold became a medical adviser for several different organisations, one of which was a charity that helped Romanian orphans suffering from HIV and AIDS. He derived great satisfaction from this work, and continued to visit the orphanage once a year, and also to give advice at other times, until he was well into his seventies. It was a way to keep in touch with his medical expertise, but with a much reduced commitment of time and energy. This arrangement gave him plenty of time to pursue his hobbies and to travel.

---

Coming to the end of your medical working life is an important transition that includes giving up your identity as a doctor, which has been an integral part of you for many years.

You may also be going through other life transitions such as retirement, moving house, loss of a partner, or children leaving home, at the same time as you decide to leave Medicine.

Although you have and will continue to have many different roles in your life, you may have found that your medical identity dominated your time and energy. So, whatever the reason for your leaving Medicine, whether it has been a planned decision to retire or resign or whether it has been forced on you because of ill health or dismissal, it is very common to experience a strong reaction to the change in your status and your lifestyle.

You may either feel as if you have been thrown on to the scrapheap of life or, in contrast, you may be over the moon about getting out of a profession which you haven't enjoyed for many years, wanting to leave but never having the courage to do so until now. You may be aware of both of these reactions. You may also be excited about the new and fresh possibilities which will be there for you if you are open to them.

Whatever initiated your decision to leave Medicine, you are very likely to go through a grieving process as you make the transition. When you move from Medicine into a world beyond, you may well experience feelings of sadness, guilt, anger and eventually acceptance and moving on, maybe into another job or a different role in your new status of retired or 'former' doctor.

You can prepare for a life after Medicine by looking at ways to deal with loss and change, grieving, retirement, growing older and change in identity and status in the community. You have to manage your personal transition not only for yourself, but also for the way others cope with it. You may be amazed at the reactions of colleagues and even friends and family when you tell them that you are planning to leave Medicine. You will be perceived differently by them, and some of them may be angry with you or jealous of your audacity in stepping into a life after Medicine.

When you are considering your life after Medicine, the following technique is very useful and also emphasises how necessary it is to know what goals you are moving towards as well as what you are moving away from. When you have those moments of doubt about whether you are doing the right thing, step back for a moment from your day-to-day concerns and in your mind's eye imagine yourself a few years in the future in the two scenarios – if you stay, and if you leave.

When you consider the latter scenario, think clearly about how life could be for you after Medicine. Then look back at yourself and recognise what you need to do now in order to have the life you want in the future. Decide what changes you need to make now. Thinking of yourself in this way may offer you a sudden realisation of what you must start right now in order to make that future possible.

Dr Copper had dreamt of taking part in the London Marathon for years, but he never got round to it. He imagined himself crossing the finishing line and hearing the cheers. Then he looked at himself now – unfit, overweight and not having started any fitness training. He knew that in order to achieve what he wanted he must make a plan to get fit over the next six months. Even though he was still working he decided that he would leave work no later than 6 pm so that he could do some training on the way home, and he also decided that he would travel to work by bicycle.

Leaving the medical profession isn't the end of the road. You may be aware of an air of excitement exuded by many people when they talk about all of the things they plan to do after leaving Medicine. However, it is a common experience to approach this new phase of your life with a mixture of expectation and apprehension about coping with less routine and the opportunities it brings to do things which you have long wanted to do. You have the option of putting your ideas into practice, so long as you are prepared to take a leap into the unknown and trust the process of change.

So why is leaving Medicine such a significant transition? If you have been part of the medical profession, the idea of breaking out of your familiar mould in order to encounter many changes in your day-to-day activities probably feels somewhat scary. However, there are new opportunities out there for whatever it is you want now in your life. All you have to do is be brave enough not only to find those opportunities but also to take them. You no longer have the excuse of not having enough time, being on call or having too many busy clinics to do whatever it is you want to do. Now you have to decide what you actually will do, and then go ahead and do it.

Transformation can seem scary, but when you leave Medicine you have the opportunity to do almost whatever you want. You might decide that you are not going to change anything and that you will keep on working as a doctor until you drop. However, this is totally unrealistic – you will change because, like it or not, this is inevitable. Change one thing and everything else will change, too. If you modify your work practice you become different in other people's eyes, they behave differently towards you and you react to them in a different way.

When you leave Medicine you have the opportunity to change what you don't like and to do more of what you really love to do. In the end, it's about attitude of mind. It's about deciding that life will be fulfilling and enjoyable even after Medicine.

Exhilaration is often the predominant feeling during that first week or two after leaving Medicine and not working. You may feel elated about leaving 'that place' and never having to be answerable to 'those people' again, and as you remember some of 'those things' which perhaps were the last straw that resulted in you deciding to stop, resign or take early retirement, you may feel quite angry about the way people behaved towards you over the years. You may remember how you gave your all and yet received very little recognition for what you did. So now you have the last laugh and they will have to manage without you, with a replacement who won't know the job as well as you! Doesn't that feel great?

Then you may begin to wonder if you will ever get into any kind of routine again. A sense of laziness may set in when you mooch around the house all day, not really wanting to do anything much, perhaps regretting that you have left Medicine and hoping that it wasn't a big mistake. It's important to develop a new schedule that is suitable for you now, so that you can enjoy the freedom of not having to be engaged in medical work any longer.

How can you keep your mind active when you give up Medicine? Challenges present themselves every day. Life after Medicine, like the rest of life, is an ongoing learning experience. Don't expect to know all the answers right away. When you know what you want you will be able to search for and find the answer. You may realise that you need to go to a professional such as a financial adviser or a solicitor if you require specialist knowledge.

You know what you want already, even if you can't describe it in detail yet, because this knowing may be quite deeply hidden in your subconscious mind. You will discover some new things about your life purpose and understand yourself a bit more as you go through your transition. There will be good days and bad ones. There will be people who give encouragement and others who don't. Keep with those who support you, and move onward to achieve what you really want in life now.

After regularly using the skills that you learned over many years while working as a doctor, you may be worried about wasting these skills when you leave Medicine. Some transferable skills will continue to be useful and some won't, and you may not use them in precisely the same way as you did before.

> **Pulsepoints**
>
> If, as a doctor, you effectively organised your day, your workspace and your life to fit in all that you needed to do, then you can apply those skills to your life after Medicine so that you can get on with the task in hand without the overwhelming effects and stress of the medical work environment.
>
> Skills that you acquired as a result of being a conscientious doctor may include:
> - being organised
> - working out plans for action
> - focusing on the task in hand
> - continuing with a task even if it takes longer than expected
> - communicating effectively
> - researching and finding options
> - planning strategies.

> **Prescription**
>
> Devise streamlined systems for getting things done in relation to your:
> - self-care
> - household tasks
> - hobbies
> - friends
> - family
> - community
> - partner.

What is important is to make a shift in your life balance, away from the stress of Medicine and towards the enjoyment of a life that you really want instead. Allow yourself more time for relaxation while also having a system in place to move your projects forward.

You are beginning a new journey into another stage of your life and you need not only plans to fulfil but also motivation and 'get up and go' to make a difference, as well as plenty of energy and enthusiasm.

Life after Medicine is a big adventure, and you are about to set out on the biggest voyage of all, so recognise the possibilities and opportunities that are there for you now. Keep calm, and while acknowledging the excitement that you feel, don't let yourself be carried away by it. In order to achieve, you need to work out your plans, draw up a timetable for action and brush away any objections that may surface in your own mind or be raised by others.

Consider carefully what you want for yourself. Develop your vision and the steps that you need to take to achieve it. To make changes you need to see what you want very clearly and then make decisions about which steps to take. Have a time frame, too, because it acts like a workplace deadline, which most people find is extremely motivating for getting things done.

You will need plenty of energy. If you don't have enough, start to look after yourself by switching to a healthy diet and taking regular exercise. Changing any habit is a powerful way to enable other things to change, too.

---

**Pulsepoints**

If fitness is something you want to achieve, or maintain, as a way to slow down the negative effects of ageing, this has to be a priority after leaving Medicine, because you may begin to suffer the side-effects of past indiscretions.

Perhaps you have started to notice some aches and pains because you haven't taken enough exercise, due to sitting in clinics and meetings for hours, or your waistline may have expanded as a result of too much hospital food.

---

**Prescription**

Start a 'get healthy' campaign. You know how important your health is, so commit to doing something about the parts that you have neglected in the past. For example:

- Get your muscles moving.
- Keep your joints flexible.
- Eat healthily.
- Drink alcohol in moderation.
- Don't smoke.

---

As you get older you will have noticed that your body isn't able to do as much as it used to do. However, regular gentle exercise is vitally important. Walking is accessible to most people. You could also consider yoga, T'ai Chi, dancing or golf. Keep moving, bending and stretching and you will slow down those inevitable body changes. Aim to achieve both a supple body and a flexible mind for your life after Medicine.

Confidence and self-belief are two vital ingredients to move you in new directions when you leave Medicine. If one or other of these is missing, you may find that life trudges on without much positive improvement. To open the doors to your new life you also need to check that you have the physical and emotional ability to look at life through new eyes, as well as the persistence to keep on trying when things don't work out the way you want them to at first.

Rather than regarding failure as the end, there is always something to be learned·from every experience. Don't give up. Be like a toddler learning to walk – he doesn't stop trying at the first fall, but instead he gets up again and continues trying until he manages to take some steps forward. You must be prepared to do this, too, when you explore new ways to live your life after Medicine. If you are lacking in confidence about your ability to do this, think of some affirmations beginning with 'I am . . .' that state whatever it is you want to achieve as if you have already succeeded. Repeat these to yourself all day long, hundreds of times, so that your subconscious mind recognises your statements as true. As a result you will find that what you affirm begins to happen. So, for example, if you keep repeating to yourself 'I am confident', this will result in a positive change in your level of confidence.

What might stop you making the changes that you want to make? Distractions can be caused by:

➤ other tasks that need to be done
➤ people who put you down with regard to what you want to do, or who make requests of you such as 'Now you've left Medicine you won't be so busy, so you will have time to do so and so for me'
➤ procrastination, which is commonplace and may be because you haven't yet clarified your destination, so you can't be clear about how to get there
➤ fear about not succeeding, especially when you have told someone about your plans.

Before you have started to implement your plans there isn't a problem, but if you fail to succeed once you have embarked upon them, are you brave enough to tell others?

In addition to learning from failure and not giving up too quickly, it's important to make an attempt, and if you don't achieve your objective having the integrity to admit that it wasn't for you, and trying something else instead. It is better to have attempted something and failed – yet also to have learned from that experience – than never to have even tried something which interests you.

In response to criticism you need to be very clear about what outcome you want. Then, keeping the big picture in mind, you will realise that it won't help if you get distracted by agreeing to do other things. If you consent too readily to do something you don't want to do, rather than what you know you want to do, then perhaps you need to re-examine your desired outcome and how strongly you want to achieve it. When you have a goal and a plan that you are passionate about, procrastination and distraction are less likely to occur. Remain very clear about how much you can move yourself towards your goals for your life after Medicine.

Draw up a plan in the form of a timetable so that you can follow a daily routine for getting the project completed. You also need to decide how to deal with distractions – for example, by saying 'Not now, but I can do it at such and such a time' – so that you have the time to do all the things you want to do.

Once you start on your journey towards change, exploration to find your life's purpose can be very exciting and rewarding. You will find that you can manage change in your life so much better once you are clear about your purpose. This is a step further than goal setting, and one which some people find quite difficult because they don't feel motivated to achieve the goals they set themselves. When you are clear about your purpose, your goals will become clearer because they are the way you can achieve that purpose – they are the steps you need to take to move towards it.

Almost anyone who has left the medical profession after many years will tell you what a major life transition this process is. For many people their whole identity is so tied up with their professional role that leaving may mean losing their identity, but that isn't necessarily so, because a person is more than their job or profession. Even while working as a doctor you have more than one role, don't you? You may be a parent, brother or sister, or son or daughter, or you may be a team member or an organiser. When you are in these roles you probably find that your identity is different, too – the way you dress, the conversations you enjoy, and so on.

When you leave Medicine you will be aligning yourself with your non-working roles much more, and you will also be developing hidden aspects of your self which have not surfaced before, perhaps because of the restrictions of the medical work environment. Being aware of your purpose helps you to decide what you will be doing during the rest of your life after Medicine.

How can you find your purpose? You may already be aware of some of the things that drive you with passion, and these may be related to your purpose. This exercise is done with pen and paper, alone or with a sympathetic friend or guide. A simple approach is as follows. Write at the bottom of a piece of paper three things you love to do or which make you feel fantastic. Starting with the first one, ask yourself 'When I . . . (whatever you started with) . . . what does that do for me?' Then reply 'It makes me . . .' and write above the first phrase what you said. Then continue asking yourself the question and writing down each answer. Eventually you will come to a stop or you may loop back to something you have said already. When that happens (and it may not be until you have about ten responses written down), go to the next thing which you love to do and repeat the process. Then do it again with number three. You will then have a sheet of paper filled with the essence of what you love to do. Look for similarities between the lists and notice any sense in your body when you read through the top words. When you feel the emotion, the excitement, as you read the words, you have found your purpose. You can begin to ask yourself 'So, in order to achieve my purpose, which is . . . , what do I need to do? How will I do it? Where? When?' And you know the 'Why?'

When you discover your purpose you will begin to realise why you find certain things so important. You will gain clarity about what you need to do and how to spend your time, and your life will take on more meaning. Once you know your purpose, look at the things which lead to it. This is also what is known as your legacy – what will be left after you have died. What do you want to leave for others to remember you by? This may be related to something creative such as painting, writing or composing, an organisation you started or sponsored, or a collection of your belongings that is donated to a museum. What will your legacy be?

Spirituality is part of who you are, whether or not you adhere to or follow a traditional religion. It is about the belief that there is a connection with something outside of yourself, which you may call God, Jehovah, Allah, The Universe, Higher Self, or anything else. You may follow the teachings of a particular religion, but even if you don't, you can still connect with your spiritual side and discover that there is part of you which is as important as your physical being. You can call this your spirituality. You may be aware of it when you are in nature and you observe phenomena of the natural world such as a beautiful sunrise or sunset. You may feel it when you see the power of the ocean and the waves crashing against the cliffs, or when you hear birds returning from their migration, or when you have climbed a mountain and are absorbing the view from the top. As a doctor, you may have been aware of this feeling when seeing a new life emerge when you were present at a birth, or while you were with someone at the moment of death, when their life force leaves their physical body.

Whatever it is that makes you aware of a power beyond yourself is your spirituality, which is beyond your physical identity and is connected to your reason for being alive. It is part of the human condition, and it's important to feel these connections on a regular basis. You can do this on your own in a way suggested, or during activities such exercise, reading, music and yoga, or anything which nurtures you and helps your body and mind to connect with your spirit.

If you have ignored this vital part of yourself in the past, remember that it is what you need for your personal well-being and for looking after body, mind and spirit.

When you consider all the various aspects of yourself that contribute to having the life you want, quality of life is hugely affected by your environment. If you have always wanted to live somewhere different, consider whether leaving Medicine can also be the time to move. Although moving house is another stress-related experience and so maybe shouldn't be done immediately, it is certainly something to be incorporated into your plans, as your environment affects the way in which you view life. What difference would it make to you if you could hear seagulls, or waves crashing on the shore, compared with the hum of motorway traffic or the screech of brakes at a main road junction? You decide. It's different for everyone. You may have had enough of moving house during specialist rotation, having to live where the job dictated rather than where you wanted to be.

Where you live depends on many things, of course, and moving to a completely different place may or may not be what you want but, since environment can also mean your personal surroundings, part of the process of moving on in life is clearing away some or all of your accumulated clutter so that you are surrounded by things you love. Clearing physical space gives room for new things to come into your life. Also, by getting rid of the encumbrances of medical work, you are indicating that you are open to something different. You really don't need to keep all those agendas or handouts from your student days, nor the huge pile of medical journals that you never got around to reading.

Whether you prefer a peaceful environment or a more noisy place to live, remember to consider both the big picture and the smaller one. Something as simple as changing the ornaments on a shelf may have a positive effect on the way you feel about life. If your home needs decorating, change the colour on the walls and you will transform your view of life, too. Throw away the clothes you will never wear again in your life after Medicine and you will have the space to acquire a new image for the next stage of your life. When the outside pleases you, your inside will delight you, too. When you re-arrange your furniture you will find a new positive perspective.

Friendships and relationships are important at all stages of your life. During your medical career, and especially when training, you may have had to move frequently and so you became adept at making new connections and friendships. These may have been primarily with colleagues, because you were far too busy to have any kind of social life at the end of the long working day. As you move into your life after Medicine, you notice changes in the way that you socialise, too. Some friendships are solid and continue throughout life, while others need to be left behind. Perhaps those you had during your medical career will no longer have the commonality of the workplace, but there are other friends to be made to go along with the new interests and activities you engage in at this time. It may be a challenge to start to make completely new friends, unrelated to the medical profession, and you may feel that you are out of practice, even though you may have been great at communicating with patients and colleagues. You may become aware of how you project your personality on to others, and you may perhaps need to adjust this somewhat.

Your relationship with your significant other – spouse or partner – is very likely to change, too, when you leave Medicine, and may be a potential cause of stress. How you cope with this may depend on the lifestyle and daily routine that you adopt. If you are at home more than you used to be, the dynamics of your relationship will change and there will need to be some time for adjustment on both sides. You should be aware of and respect each other's need for space (both physical and emotional). Unless you worked together, you will be in each other's company for far longer than you have been for years. It is an opportunity to get to know each other again and to come to terms with shared and differing interests, so that you have time together and time apart, too.

---

Dr Brass, a retired GP, found it difficult to accept that his wife still went out to work as a health visitor. She found his regular phone calls to ask her when she would be getting home very upsetting. Eventually he obtained some work as a medical adviser to a television company, and found that having at least some small routine in his day was helpful. His wife encouraged him to learn some simple cooking skills, something he had neglected to develop while working at his busy job, so that he could help her by having a meal ready when she came back from work.

---

Happiness is an overwhelming priority for most people, and particularly at this time when you may be questioning your decision to leave Medicine. When you feel happy, contented and fulfilled, you will know that you made the right choice. However, during times of uncertainty a sense of unhappiness may overwhelm you, so it is important to do whatever you can to be as happy as possible most of the time.

How will you go about deciding what to do and how to go ahead and start taking some definite action towards achieving what you want? Too many people say 'One day I'll do so and so,' yet they never actually get around to doing any of it. If you want the satisfaction of a life well lived and are clear about what you want to accomplish during the rest of your life, make a commitment to make a start.

It is said that new habits need to be repeated at least 21 times to fix them into the subconscious mind, so it will be small things repeated day by day that make a difference to your big picture. Pick something which is different from your normal routine. Changing any habit tends to make it easier to change others. If you find it difficult to start, try something apparently unconnected. For example, change what you eat for breakfast or the style or colour of clothes that you wear, and notice what happens.

You can begin to experience a sense of serenity when you go with the flow, and things will eventually start to move forward. In the end it depends on you, your preparatory work, the steps that you decide to take initially and your passion to get ready for a wonderful, exciting and rewarding life after Medicine.

Be inspired, motivated and push yourself forward out of your old life and into a new one. Prepare yourself fully and get ready for a great life after Medicine. Continue to daydream as you may have done for years, although now the time has come to transform the dream into your reality.

➤ Are you ready to take the dream out of your head and your imagination into the world outside?

➤ Are you ready to let others know what it is you've been longing for during those years of medical work, when perhaps the thoughts about leaving and what you would have time to do kept you going through hours of fatigue and being overwhelmed?

Now is the time for your ideas to take precedence. There are no managers or government targets to satisfy now, and no more work-related deadlines. You are your own boss and you can do whatever you want.

How will you start to develop the new way of life that you are about to begin? You have the dream, but now you must plan how to translate this into some kind of reality. You may once more need to have your own deadlines and be accountable to yourself or to someone you choose to support you, but you can decide by when you want to achieve them and to whom you will be responsible. Set a realistic date by which you want to achieve the whole dream, and then break it down into smaller chunks so that week by week you can achieve sensible amounts. Plan what you will do each day to move the dream closer to achievement. Then, little by little, change will start to happen. Even five or ten minutes each day will move things forward. Many people find this is a more effective way to make progress than planning to do a huge amount in one day. You can do small amounts of several jobs each day, or set aside a larger block of time to complete one task fully. You could change activities every half an hour, from sitting still to moving around, or you may find allocating a whole day to something suits your personality better. That's fine so long as you actually do it, as too many people have this intention but don't use a full day to complete a task.

Flow is the way to go. Water finds its own level. When you go with your flow you will find the life you want. However, you need to have plans, too, otherwise you may say that you are going with the flow when in fact you are becoming a couch potato. You need to have a timetable that may be more fluid than the one you had to follow as a doctor. Starting every day with absolutely no idea of what you are going to do is unlikely to result in achieving your dreams and your purpose. Yes, you can have wonderful dreams of what you would like, but when you plan specifically how to take them forward you will find that time will pass more quickly than you could possibly imagine. You don't have unlimited time – you have the time you have, full stop. You don't know what the future may bring you. You don't know how long it may be before you are unable to do the things you want to do. So take the reins to your new life and ride it the way you want it to go. When it goes slightly off course, as it will inevitably do from time to time, you have to decide whether to explore another new path for a while and then pull yourself back to the one you were on before, or whether the new path seems to be a better one to follow. That's OK, too, because it's fine to change direction so long as you realise that you no longer have forever, so go along the new path, explore other possibilities, but then ask yourself how or if these will help you to fulfil your purpose, your ambition and what you really want to achieve above all else.

You need a schedule to keep you on some kind of track so that when you look back week by week or month by month you can see that you are making progress, and it helps if you can approach all of this with a lightness of heart and a lightness of step and emotion. You need clarity about where your passion lies, and you should be able to move forward towards it without, if possible, harming or upsetting others. Communicate, explain and make every challenge into a learning experience to help you to achieve your goal.

Explore all of the potential that you have ahead of you when you leave Medicine, whatever might be fun to do, and then do it. Don't limit yourself to the things you always do, or to what people expect of you, but instead surprise them and yourself by doing something unexpected and different. You can enjoy almost anything now that you are no longer answerable to your hospital, your practice, managers, chief executive, or the work schedules which have bound you for so long. Of course you will have certain limits, and don't imagine that you could do something which is physically beyond your capabilities, for example. However, too many people curb their attempts because they believe that it is impossible because of their age, body build or the type of person they are.

---

### Pulsepoints

Whatever you dream of, make the plan, write the steps in your diary and then take the action required. If it's a one-off activity, just do it. If it's a larger project, plan and make your own deadline and schedule to follow. Take it one step at a time, remembering that your steps can be as large or as small as you wish, as long as you take them so that you will move forward into the life you want. Having a sense of humour is optional, but it helps! Learning new ways to do things is part of the great excitement waiting for you when you leave Medicine. You have reached this stage of your life having developed many skills in relation to your medical work, and now you can adapt these skills to your new life and also have fun exploring and learning new ways to use them. Perhaps there are specific skills that you want to learn.

> **Prescription**
>
> Find out about:
> - your local adult education centre and what it has to offer. Perhaps you can offer your skills to others. It's very rewarding at the end of a long career to be able to mentor others who are just starting out
> - the University of the Third Age and how you can learn and teach others, because teaching is as useful as learning. As you teach you also learn. The questions you are asked will make you aware of how things change (and perhaps make you come to terms with the fact that it really was time to leave Medicine)
> - developing talents which you may have kept suppressed for years. Perhaps you have hidden your creative abilities. Pick up a paintbrush or a piece of charcoal and find out what happens. Maybe you have always wanted to write poetry or a novel, so get started and let the ideas flow. You can learn the basics and meet others with the same passions as you, and then you have permission to explore your creativity to the full.

Plan your day. Plan your week. Plan your month. Not in a rigid way like a work schedule, but in a fluid way that allows some flexibility. Don't let yourself become an inactive person who spends too much time sitting and doing very little.

It may be a temptation, when you no longer have the routine of work, to sit around and watch television and eat crisps all day, but this isn't the way to have a rewarding life after Medicine. Instead, what you have to do now that you have the time to plan your days is to connect with your passion and then, with the enthusiasm you generate from thinking about what it is that fires you up, start doing something differently. Devise a strategy that will, step by manageable step, move you from where you are now to where you want to be at some specified date in the future.

Remember that it is not just the final accomplishment that matters. It is working out how you can get from here to there, and what steps you have to take to move yourself. When you do this you won't be lazy any more because your excitement gives you the energy to move yourself forward and achieve what you want, and you will be able to do this by letting go of things you did which you no longer have to do now, or which you no longer have to do so often. Share the tasks which absolutely have to be done with your partner or with other members of your family. Tell them that you won't be quite so available as they would perhaps like you to be!

Prioritise what you have to do so that you don't become overwhelmed as you did when you were working. You don't have to do everything, but you need to decide what absolutely has to be done today, what can be done gradually, starting today, and what need not be done at all. You may choose to spend some of your day doing things such as watching television, when there are other more important things to do, but you could decide not to waste time in this way any more. Notice what distracts you from the task in hand, and take steps to decide how to deal with this. If your neighbour turns up uninvited and expecting coffee and a chat, explain that it is not convenient at the moment, and suggest a time that is suitable for you.

You could:

➤ make a timetable, so you have a rough idea of what you plan to do each day

➤ divide your time between different types of tasks so that you can vary what you do every hour

➤ do something physical and then something that involves sitting at your computer

➤ recognise that you don't have to finish one task completely before you do part of another, because the very process of starting something makes it easier to return to it later and continue where you left off.

Achievement is wonderful, but the journey towards it can be satisfying, too. When you know what you are passionate about, then you can find the time to take the steps towards it. The big goal, the vision, your purpose, will all drive your motivation and enable you to look at what options you have to reach it. If you feel stuck in a rut, lacking the driving force to proceed, or are fed up with people being cynical about your ability to reach your goal, or are using the excuse of not having the time to do something which would move you towards the life you want, then think again. Is it truly what you want? Can you imagine what it would be like to live the life you imagine? Picture the scene, and imagine yourself there. Does thinking about it fill you with excitement or dread? Perhaps you need to reconsider exactly what you want, and if what you want is the same as what you previously decided, relax and brainstorm as many ideas as possible of all the ways to move forward.

Strange though it may seem, if you keep asking yourself 'How else could I achieve that?' you will think of lots of other ways. Once you obtain clarity about what you truly want, you will have the motivation to take the steps that are necessary.

# CHAPTER 8

# Time for a fresh start?

Leaving Medicine is a time to re-assess, to come to terms with the fact that you no longer have for ever to achieve what you want and make sure that you do something now. It's about recognising your passage through life and your eventual mortality, accepting what you can and can't do and deciding to achieve what your heart desires before it's too late. Even if you have been forced to leave Medicine through circumstances beyond your control, that doesn't mean it's depressing, a time to sit back and fall into a heap in the corner, or raise your hands and drop your head in a resigned sort of a way and do absolutely nothing. No, it's an opportunity to recognise that, whatever your age, you can do something more in line with your dreams.

**Pulsepoints**

Looking after your body, mind and spirit is an absolutely vital part of having a balanced and fulfilled life after Medicine.

**Prescription**

Think about your priorities for your own health and well-being, and draw up a chart for yourself. Put it in a prominent position and challenge yourself to tick all the boxes on your chart every day for the next three weeks. It may be difficult at first, but if you persist you will find that most of those habits will become second nature to you.

Dr Plum knew what he had to do, but found it a challenge to take action. So to motivate himself he made a chart listing the various activities he had decided to do in order to have more balance and improve his health and well-being in his life after Medicine. Each day he ticked what he had managed to do that day. His list included the following: walk for 30 minutes, drink two litres of water, eat five portions of fruit and vegetables, do yoga, read three chapters of a novel, limit alcohol intake to two glasses of wine or less.

Years ago, people strongly believed that 'once a doctor, always a doctor' – that Medicine was a vocation and you had to stick it out to the end, however much you wanted to do something else. However, if contrary to all the advice you were given about what a bad thing it would be to leave, you chose to do so, then you would be seen as a failure and people would feel sorry for you.

Even at the official retirement age you would have a party, be given a present and good wishes from your work colleagues and then be sent off to laze about and do nothing, although you would be expected to be on a committee or two, and perhaps be called from time to time to 'keep your hand in' by doing some locums. You would have retained your identity and status as a doctor, too. Colleagues would joke about wishing that they too could spend all day playing golf or doing nothing all day, and that would be it. You would probably have done exactly that, in between occasional meetings and locums – eaten too much, maybe drunk too much, exercised too little and eventually come to an early end. Not a very happy picture, is it?

Things are very different these days. There are young doctors considering leaving the profession, and many actually doing so. They are not prepared to put up with the long hours required of them when doing so substantially impairs their quality of life. More doctors have family responsibilities and want to be there for their children and partner. This attitude was very much frowned upon in the past. Doctors were compelled to devote all their time and energy to their work, and were not expected to let the challenges of childcare interfere with their work schedules.

I once talked to my consultant about my children having chickenpox and how unhappy I was about leaving them in the care of a young au pair. She told me that she had five children, always worked full time, employed a live-in nanny and would never even contemplate taking time off work to look after her children.

---

Doctors nowadays are not prepared to hand over the full-time responsibility of childcare completely.

---

Dr Ruby, an orthopaedic surgeon, was told off by his consultant when he looked after his children while his GP wife did an afternoon surgery. The time was designated 'research time' for him, and he did this work later in the evening. He was told that 'Your wife shouldn't have to work, but if she chooses to do so then she must find her own childcare.'

---

Maybe you chose to leave Medicine before the statutory retirement age, or were made redundant, or found that you could no longer cope with the stress of the work, or had a physical or mental health problem which forced you to take early retirement. Perhaps you decided to leave Medicine in order to satisfy a lifelong wish to do something entirely different, possibly involving connecting with your creativity, and you reached a point in your life when you realised that you could afford to give up your medical salary and that you had earned enough to cover your day-to-day needs for the next part of your life.

It is challenging and can be rather daunting to enter any new phase of life, because dealing with transition and change will have its ups and downs. When you are preparing to leave Medicine, it helps if you are fully prepared for the emotional rollercoaster that you may experience.

Perhaps you have been telling people for years about all the things you would do if you weren't so busy. You would have time to catch up and do all those jobs you've been putting off for years.

On the other hand, you may choose not to leave, but instead adapt your medical work in a way that allows you to have a better work–life balance, so that you have the time to get involved in other interests outside medical work. If you have been thinking about change for some time, but have not actually done anything, then the first strategy for preparing yourself for action is to recognise that you can do whatever you set your mind to (well, almost anything).

> **Pulsepoints**
>
> Leaving Medicine is a time to come to terms with how you may be sabotaging yourself regularly by making all kinds of assumptions about your own abilities, what you want to do, how others might react to you doing certain things and the compromises that you therefore believe you have to make, even if these result in not doing even part of what you want to do.

> **Prescription**
>
> Separate assumptions from reality. Start this process by asking the following questions:
> * What evidence is there for making this assumption?
> * How do I know how he or she will react?
> * How do I know what life will be like if I do the other?

It's very common to have ideas about other people and the way they may react to a certain situation, when in fact all that these ideas are based on is a guess, without any evidence. Assumptions without evidence are often used as a reason for not doing something. They are excuses that you make to yourself about why the course of action that you are apprehensive about might not, after all, be suitable.

When you enter this new phase of your life – your life after Medicine – the very first step is to mentally prepare yourself for 'take-off.' Then you can move on to the subsequent steps, but only then. What do you have to do to move smoothly and glide onwards and upwards? Look at the statements below, and if you agree with any of them, you will benefit from the suggestions in this book.

➤ Your life seems to be completely out of balance at the moment.
➤ You wonder how you will cope without the routines of work.
➤ You are willing to explore the idea of doing something different.
➤ You have neglected your health and well-being.
➤ You want to enjoy a life after Medicine.
➤ You want more time for friends and family.
➤ You would like to spend more quality time with your partner.
➤ You have the energy, motivation and enthusiasm to change.
➤ You are ready to look after yourself more effectively.

# CHAPTER 9

# A balanced life

There are three important steps you must take to make a smooth transition between Medicine and the rest of your life. You need to **decide, organise** and **accomplish.**

First, **decide** what you want for your life after Medicine. Do you already know what your goals are for a fulfilled and happy life after Medicine, or are you only thinking about leaving behind the stress of the medical workload? Until you know what you want rather than what you don't want, it will be difficult to move forward positively in your life.

---

**Pulsepoints**

Setting clear goals about your desired life after Medicine is essential. Although you may say that you want the transition to be a smooth one, so that you hardly notice any negative effects of leaving the medical profession behind, have you identified clearly what that actually means for you?

---

> **Prescription**
>
> In order to discover what having a perfect transition from Medicine means to you, ask yourself the following questions:
> - Do you believe you can deal emotionally and physically with the change that you are considering?
> - Do you dread leaving Medicine so much that you might decide to carry on doing your own locum?
> - Do you worry that work has filled your days, months and years so completely that you hardly have any other interests?
> - Are you afraid of being bored?
> - Do you lack the confidence to get yourself to the place where you can do what you want?

You have had a fairly structured life for years, even allowing for the unexpected emergencies. You know the way things are organised for medical work – the clinics, surgeries and on-call duties – and even though there were emergencies to deal with, there was still a routine and a certain predictability. You had an expectation of how your days would be filled, and even though there were varying workloads and you knew they would generally be large, you usually knew what might happen within that work context.

Then from one day to the next your agenda changes and you want to:

➤ read all the books which have been piling up, waiting for when you have some spare time, because it would be wonderful to read on a regular basis, maybe join a readers' group and discuss your opinions about the various books

➤ see your children, grandchildren or other relatives more often because they want to get to know you better

➤ be able to go to the cinema each week, and see all the latest films as they are released instead of on television several years later

➤ get fitter by walking more, running or swimming regularly, joining a yoga class or playing golf

➤ get your photos sorted out before you become too old to remember when and where they were taken

➤ start a business

➤ upgrade your computer skills

➤ learn a new language.

There will no longer be any excuses because when you are very clear about your desired outcome, you will find it easy to make big steps into your desired life after Medicine.

As you plan for your new phase of life, you may be feeling a bit wobbly, because you are fed up with the lack of balance in your life and you have told yourself that enough is enough.

Years of trying to be all things to all people may have seemed rather like trying to balance a beam horizontally on a fulcrum, when it naturally wants to tip either one way or the other. When this happens, you may feel overwhelmed by all the things there are to do one day, and then too lazy to do anything at all at other times. That's what it's like being a doctor, and when you leave you no longer have to keep to a tight schedule – day in, day out – while at the same time dealing with emergencies and other responsibilities. Over the years this lack of balance amounts to not much of a life if it continues week in, week out and you never get to do all the exciting things you've been promising yourself you would do one day. Not only is it not much of a life, but it is not good for your personal, emotional and physical health and well-being, or for your personal relationships.

---

After she left Medicine, Dr Stone thought that she should do her house-work in order to save money, as she was earning less. However, she found it so stressful and boring that eventually she decided it was worth the cost of employing a cleaner to relieve her stress.

---

Keep in your mind the picture of the beam balanced on a fulcrum as you become more aware of when it tips too much to one side or the other, and thus your need to do something to get it back to some kind of equilibrium if you want your life to be more balanced, with your needs addressed.

**Pulsepoints**

Watch carefully to see whether your life keeps becoming out of balance by falling towards the needs and demands of your partner, friends or family, and rarely falling to the side of what you want to do. It is likely to do this if you don't address your own needs for health and well-being by being clear and asking for what you actually want – hence the importance of goal setting. It's so simple to keep on doing what you have always done. Perhaps you complain and groan but then carry on as before. It's easier to strike a balance when you recognise what it is that is pulling you one way, and compare this with what is pulling you the other way.

**Prescription**

- Make a list of five things which pull you away from the life you want.
- List five things which would push you towards a more balanced life.
- Draw pictures of a beam or a see-saw sloping down one way, sloping down the other, and horizontal. Note on each diagram what pushes you out of balance one way or the other.
- Decide how friends, family, partner and community affect your life balance.

**Pulsepoints**

To work out your strategy for change, make sure that you express your desired outcome in positive terms, rather than by saying what you don't want.

**Prescription**

Create some affirmations which express what you want to achieve as if you have already achieved it. For example, instead of saying 'I wish I had a better life than this', you could say 'I have a wonderful life. I have plenty of time to do all the things I want to do.'

You have to decide what your perfect life after Medicine would be for you, and be really clear about what it would look like, sound like and feel like, so that you can live it.

---

Dr Leaf knew that he wanted to be a professional photographer when he stopped working as a doctor. At first he found the change of lifestyle very challenging, but he was willing to try visualisation. He gradually mastered the technique, which is rather like daydreaming. He could imagine himself lying on his front taking wonderful pictures on wildlife safaris, he heard people praising his dramatic photos, and he felt the thrill of making a success of this new career. Doing this motivated him to take a course in professional photography and explore ways to take his desired new life forward. This included remaining very focused and not being distracted from his aim by his friends and family doubting his ability to make a success of this new venture by telling him that he shouldn't have left Medicine.

---

### Pulsepoints

When these things are clear and you see yourself as you would like to be in your life after Medicine, you will be ready to move towards creating that life.

If you write down your goals you are more likely to succeed.

### Prescription

For each goal, write down three smaller steps that you will need to take to reach it. In your diary, note the steps and when you will make time to do them. Write your goals for the next three months and the dates by when you want to achieve them.

Secondly, **organise** your time more effectively by defining the various 'compartments' of your day and of your life. For example, you may have parts of your day which are used for:

➤ domestic tasks
➤ hobbies
➤ keeping fit
➤ your children

➤ your partner
➤ your friends and family
➤ the community
➤ spiritual connection.

---

**Pulsepoints**

Think about what you are planning for your life after Medicine and how to make it more balanced than it was when you were a doctor, even though you may not have been very good at doing this in the past.

---

**Prescription**

- List all the tasks that you don't enjoy and decide what to delegate.
- Decide which of these habits don't actually have to be done at all.
- Devise strategies for doing things more efficiently.
- Let go of checking and re-checking and trust your ability to do a good job first time around.

---

Finally, **accomplish** and achieve whatever you have decided is your desired outcome and the steps you will take. The next thing is to take that first step. It sounds easy, doesn't it? If you have done this before but got stuck, this may be because the first step you thought of was too big.

---

Dr Flower wanted to travel when he left Medicine. He decided to apply to be a medical officer with a company that organised charity treks in Namibia. The first step was to contact the company and request an application form. The second step was to fill in the form and send it off. The third step was to attend an interview. The step before the first step was to contact the person already doing the job and find out the pros and cons of doing the job so that he could make an informed decision about it.

---

Do you have a problem related to the way you manage time? Whether you like it or not, time is the currency that you need for making the changes you want. You have to discover new ways to free up more time. A good way is to start to say 'no' more often. Say it when someone asks you to do an extra bit of a task because 'everyone else is far too busy.' Unless you are able to do the thing immediately, just say no. In this way you will complete your daily tasks and then have time to take the first steps towards your new life! What will you say no to now? What is preventing you from doing what you want? Is it because of:

➤ where you have to be
➤ what you might have to do
➤ the need to acquire some more skills
➤ lack of congruence with your beliefs and values
➤ conflict with who you are
➤ lack of congruence with your life's purpose?

Perhaps you feel quite scared about setting out to do something different, because this will initiate a series of changes which include becoming someone else. When you change, so do other people who connect and interact with you. However, when you finally, bravely, take that step it's a common experience to find that it isn't as frightening as you thought it would be. Generally, people are surprised at how much better they feel once they start, and then the rest becomes much easier, too. The benefits of initiating change for your life after Medicine are huge. Life will be different, so prepare for it and make it the way you want it to be instead of just letting it happen.

# CHAPTER 10

# Facing change

What many hard-working doctors like you find most challenging about leaving Medicine and trying to achieve the life they desire is trying to please everyone. Because of these attitudes you, too, may find it very difficult to say no.

During your years of medical work you were likely to have been bombarded by requests to do this task, sort out that problem, answer telephone calls, give an opinion about a situation, and all of this while you were trying to get through your day and attempting to concentrate on the matter in hand. These distractions drained your energy, were time consuming, made your life less and less balanced, and caused you to feel frustrated and exhausted. Your life after Medicine can be so different from that if you allow it to be.

At first, when you leave Medicine, you may want to do nothing until you discover some new found energy, and then you may wonder whether you can do all that you want to do during the rest of your life. There is so much opportunity, and so many things in which to be involved.

The need to look after yourself may have taken a back seat while you were a busy doctor. Like many doctors you might have been a perfectionist, and to achieve this you kept on going even when you were hungry, exhausted, and hadn't done anything except work and sleep for days on end. You might have forgotten the importance of self-care or not been able to spend any time addressing this.

Maybe for the last few years you have put your own needs aside and let the demands of your work take over your life. You knew, deep down, that this was not an acceptable state of affairs, but you carried on because you believed that you had no choice. The people who had the power to make a difference were as stressed as you were.

However, now that you are starting a life after Medicine, you really do need to eat proper food, get enough sleep and take plenty of exercise, because your health and well-being depend on you looking after yourself properly. A great life after Medicine depends on you recognising the importance of self-care.

Try thinking about your life from the perspective of an outsider. What would they see that you could change for the better?

Start to recognise your own needs as much as those of others, and notice how little you address them. Looking after your body, mind and spirit is vital. Everyone, including you, must set aside time for rest and relaxation. Acknowledge that you have permission to do this, in addition to connecting with friends and family, having a relationship, enjoying hobbies, playing an instrument, singing in a choir, or doing whatever else excites you. When you start to look after yourself much better, you will find that you begin to say no to things you don't want to do any more, because that is what you can do in your life after Medicine. When someone makes demands on you or your time, you need to recognise that there has to be some give and take. You can say 'No, I'm sorry, I can't – I have other things to do at that time.' There is no need to go into all the details, just say no, and perhaps suggest a more mutually convenient time if it's something you really want to do, as it's virtually impossible to be perfect, and 'good enough' will do.

**Pulsepoints**

If you want to do something which reaches your body, mind and spirit, try yoga. It helps you to relax and connect with your breath, and it exercises your body. You may also enjoy T'ai Chi, exercising in the gym, swimming or running. All of these help activities improve your fitness but also have an effect on your well-being, and you may notice improvements in the way you experience life, too. When you exercise regularly, your mind and spirit benefit as well as your body.

**Prescription**

Read all those books that you've been meaning to read for ages.
Even half an hour once a week will be good. Then you can:
- learn what you've always wanted to learn
- exercise your brain with crosswords or Sudoku
- nurture your spirit by connecting with formal or informal religion, or by connecting with nature and the changing seasons
- not let the challenges stop you
- list your challenges to having the life you want after Medicine
- decide how you can overcome these challenges one by one.

# CHAPTER 11

# Secrets of change

Before your proposed change, it is useful to have a conversation with three parts of yourself – dreamer, critic and realist, or with others in those roles. The dreamer has all the wonderful ideas, the critic thinks of everything which might go wrong, and the realist works out the practical ways to achieve the dream, taking into account what the critic has said.

Stand in different parts of the room designated 'dreamer', 'realist' and 'critic', and as you go to each area, ask yourself to consider your situation in the appropriate role. Notice how just by moving to a different place your perception of the situation can change. Have a conversation with these three different parts of yourself and decide if and how to take the project forward in a sensible way.

A little known secret about change is that when you start following your dream you are likely to experience a series of stages, known as the 'hero's journey' (described by Joseph Campbell). You may encounter some very briefly, and others for longer. Reflect on the journeys of change that you have made during your life and how you experienced them. At any one time you might be on several journeys each at a different stage. You may be just starting a new journey, feel stuck on one you started some time ago, or notice that you have recently completed another.

First there is 'the call' – the time when you just know something has to change. You know things can't carry on as they are. The call may be:

➤ a strong feeling or emotion that you have about your present situation

➤ what you hear from others about how things might get worse

➤ how you see yourself in the future if things carry on as they are.

Make a list of some calls you have at the moment or have had in the past (whether or not they have resulted in any change). They may be things about which you say to yourself 'One day I want to do so and so' or 'When I'm not so busy I plan to go to such and such a place.' You have a choice as to whether or not to answer the call, however it presents itself to you. Many people ignore or try to ignore it, so it goes away for a while and then comes back to nag them again.

Eventually you decide to answer this call, and to do this you set out on your metaphorical 'hero's journey.'

As you start the journey for change, you will meet many different people, the best of whom are those who support and encourage you on your way and tell you how interesting and exciting your journey appears to be. They may be friends, family, colleagues, or a mentor or coach. On the other hand, there are also those people who tell you that you have made a big mistake and should definitely go back to where you were. Both of these are very valuable so long as you balance their comments with what you really want to do. Get support from the former and travel some of your way with them, but move away from the latter and remain determined to continue your personal journey for change.

Don't be put off by the critics, but listen to them and find a realistic answer to their criticisms. Then, with these things in mind, keep going. Keep your dream alive, and your vision, your goal in view. Find the people who support and encourage you, because you will need them when you reach the next stage of your journey.

Just as you think everything is going well you reach the 'wilderness', or find yourself 'in the belly of a whale', when you strongly believe that the critics were right and you shouldn't have set out on this journey of change. You may feel terrible and don't know how to get out of what you started, as you are now convinced that it was a big mistake. Hang in there, and be reassured that this is part of the process of change. Focus on your goal and look for ways to move onward away from this stage. At this time some suitable support can also be valuable.

Eventually you will find your way out of the 'inhospitable surroundings' and can move towards your vision once more.

Finally, at last, you reach the goal you wanted so much. Then you might recognise things about it, and where you are, as strangely familiar. You may have travelled far physically and emotionally, but have found your dream not far from where you started from. If you had only realised this you might not have needed to make such a traumatic journey to reach it. This is known as 'the return.' It's the archetypal story of going around the world to find the pot of gold in your own back yard.

Achieving your goal means that you and your life are still the same, but with significant differences because you have been on a journey of self-discovery to get there. You were able to change, but perhaps you hadn't previously recognised that what you wanted was significantly connected to something you were already doing, or that was in your life already.

Where are you in your 'hero's journey'? What is stopping you from moving onward? What rocks are blocking your way forward and how will you move them?

# CHAPTER 12

# Failing to have a fulfilling life after Medicine

There are several possible reasons for lack of success in achieving the life you really want after Medicine. Be aware of them so that you don't let them spoil your chances of achieving the life you want.

## STRIVING FOR PERFECTION

Perhaps one of the main reasons why people fail to have the life they want after Medicine is because of an overwhelming desire for perfection. Be realistic – however hard you try, it may not be possible to have an 100 per cent perfect life after Medicine, even if you follow all the suggestions in this book.

What is the reason for this? It is because life has a habit of happening and things don't always work out the way you hope they will. However well you plan your day, there will be times when you can't do everything you hoped to do. Be like a tree blowing in the wind – be flexible so that you don't break under the strain. When things 'hit' you, go with the flow, adapt and adjust, and then get back on course as soon as you can.

It really is OK to be 'good enough'. This means being as competent as you possibly can be while acknowledging that things can and do go wrong and they are not necessarily anything to do with you.

## FORGETTING ABOUT THE WHEEL OF LIFE

There's more to leaving Medicine than either doing nothing or doing too much, but certain aspects of the transition are vital and you should remember to address them without fail every day. Vital areas of life have been represented as a wheel with segments known as the 'wheel of life.' You can have a visual representation of the balance in your life by noticing where your sense of fulfilment or satisfaction is in relation to the centre (= 0) and the rim (= 10) of the wheel, and being aware of and looking after these will help you to live a more fully balanced life. These include:

➤ self-care
➤ friends and family
➤ partner
➤ spirituality
➤ community
➤ fun
➤ money
➤ work (paid or voluntary).

What I have found when I have been coaching doctors over the last few years is that when they start to work with me, one of the commonest problems is not having time for anything outside of work. Within a few sessions of coaching they make a huge shift and are able to plan their day more effectively and efficiently, delegate much more, and decide to stop doing some things. The outcome of all of this is a new-found ability to leave work on time, a greater recognition of the importance of self-care, an increase in the amount of exercise and the rediscovery of long forgotten hobbies. Stress levels fall and quality of life improves. By delegating or by stopping doing some things they free up time to do what they really want to do.

## LACK OF NON-JUDGMENTAL SUPPORT

Another reason for failure to achieve your ideal life after Medicine may be because you try to do it all yourself. You fail to find support and motivation, because you may not realise how powerful it can be to have someone to talk to, bounce ideas off and be accountable to. This support needs to be non-judgmental and from a person you respect. This might be your partner or a member of your family, but be careful because often they are too close to give an objective view on what you want to discuss, especially if it involves what they see as unfavourable changes for themselves. They may be biased about you doing some things rather than others, so the conclusion you reach after talking to them may be what they think is best for you, rather than what you want to do. A friend who is going through a similar transition can be useful, but they may try to influence you as a result of their own experience. Even if it seems similar, your circumstances may be quite different, so what you want to do may also be very different. Working with a life coach or a mentor can be a useful source of support.

## LACK OF CLARITY ABOUT DESIRED OUTCOME

If you don't know where you are going, how will you know when you've got there? Not having clear desired goals is another reason why people fail. You need a plan, and you should make your desired outcome into a SMART goal:

➤ State your goal in precise terms. If you say 'I want to be happy', explain what that will mean to you. When you are happy, what will you do? What will you wear? How will you walk and talk?

➤ How will others know that you have reached your goal? What is measurable?

➤ What will they notice about you that is different? Is what you want something that you can achieve?

➤ Is it a realistic goal for you?

➤ When will you aim to achieve it? Don't just promise 'next year some time', but specify the time – for example, 'by the end of March.'

## FAILURE TO UNDERSTAND THE HIERARCHY OF NEEDS

Maslow represented human needs in the form of a pyramid or triangle, with basic physiological needs at its base and 'self-actualisation' at the top. He suggested that you have to fulfil your basic needs before you can move on to higher needs. Therefore expecting huge changes to take place in your life when you aren't eating properly or have nowhere to live is unrealistic. Look after yourself first, learn what you need to learn, teach others and spread your knowledge. Then and only then will you be in the right place to do the higher things which will have an influence on the 'big picture' and help the world be a better place. Maslow suggests that you can't change the world if you have a rumbling stomach. You have to start with the basics of looking after your physiological and shelter needs before you can achieve 'self-actualisation.'

So it is important to:
➤ eat a healthy diet, with plenty of fruit and vegetables, protein and complex carbohydrates
➤ take regular exercise to keep your body, including your heart, healthy
➤ take time to relax or to meditate or connect with nature so that you feed your spirit as well as your body
➤ look after your own needs
➤ be pro-active about self-care to raise your self-esteem and self-confidence.

## NOT UNDERSTANDING LOGICAL LEVELS

Rather like Maslow's hierarchy of needs, you can look at a situation or challenge in relation to its 'logical levels', as described by Robert Dilts. If you feel stuck about something, it is possible to identify where or what the block is and how to resolve the issue by looking at the following:
➤ environment (where?)
➤ behaviour (what?)
➤ capability (how?)
➤ beliefs and values (why?)
➤ identity (who?)
➤ beyond identity (what for?).

Think of each of these in relation to yourself as you prepare for a life after Medicine. As you consider each level in relation to your desired life, you may gain some understanding of where the problem lies. You will find that your perspective is enhanced by standing in a different place as you do this. Rather like walking forward on stepping stones, you can close your eyes and say to yourself 'I'm thinking about environment. What, if anything, do I need to do to improve this in relation to my goals?'

Let any insights enter your mind and write them in your notebook. Take time to do this. Then take a step forward and ask yourself how your behaviour needs to change in order to achieve your goal. Take another step forward and ask whether you can do this yourself or whether you need to acquire some new skills. This relates to your capability to achieve what you want to do. Take one step further and you are in the place to consider your beliefs and values with regard to what you want to achieve and whether these need to change. Take another step to ask 'Who am I? Am I the sort of person who can accomplish what I want?' Finally, ask 'What is my purpose in life? Why am I here?' From that place you can move back through the steps and re-think what each means to you. So you move from beyond identity to identity, from there to beliefs and values, then to your capability and your behaviour, and finally to environment. Then take some time to think about the insights you have gained about your life, what you want and how to do it. Once you have more clarity, go ahead and take the actions that you have to take and start to make a difference to your life.

# CHAPTER 13

# A successful life after Medicine

Here are the key points for a successful life after Medicine.

➤ Decide what you want to achieve, by setting clear goals or outcomes.

➤ List as many options as you can think of which could lead to your goal, however crazy they might be, because even those may have something which might indicate a way for you to move forward.

➤ Think of even more options.

➤ Pick one or two options and work on them. You will either progress towards your goal or be clearer about what is not going to be the solution.

➤ Be open to trying an option which at first seems less viable. Although it may not be the way forward, there may be an element of it which you can combine with another option.

➤ Draw a mind map to enable you to discover what might be involved in following one or other of your options.

➤ Use your mind map to make connections and work out whether any of these could have a practical use.

➤ Decide where and when to make a start.

➤ Decide where and when you will achieve what you want.

➤ Think about how your behaviour will change when you reach your goal.

➤ Start to change your current behaviour to be more as it will be.

➤ Define what you need to learn.

➤ Decide whether you need formal or informal training and how to achieve this.

➤ Recognise, realistically, by when you are capable of achieving what you want.

➤ Recognise whether what you want to do is congruent with your values.

➤ Know what is important for you, and beware of doing things solely because others want this for you.

➤ Know whether you are someone who keeps to your plans.

➤ Decide who can support you.

➤ Change your perception of who you are by using positive affirmations, such as 'I always achieve what I want' or 'I am confident.'

➤ Be clear about what you want to do as part of your 'big picture' of what you want to achieve in your lifetime, and whether this will be part of your legacy.

# CHAPTER 14

# Resources

➤ Further information: www.lifeaftermedicine.co.uk/resources
➤ Follow Julia Cameron's suggestions in her book *The Artist's Way*:
- Write 'morning pages', which consist of about three pages of flow-of-consciousness writing, just letting the pen write whatever it wants to write about the way you are feeling, what has been good about the day, what has been challenging, what you learned, and how you would do some of those things differently next time.
- Go on an 'artist's date'. Decide on something you really want to do and when you will do it. This is something you do just for yourself and by yourself. It might consist of visiting a place you want to visit or curling up in an armchair and reading a good book. It is something just for you, and you must plan when you will do it each week and make it a definite commitment.

## RECOMMENDED BOOKS AND REFERENCES

Buzan T, Keene R. *The Age Heresy.* London: Ebury Press; 1996.
Cameron J. *The Artist's Way.* London: Pan Books; 1995.
Campbell J. *The Hero's Journey.* Novato, CA: New World Library; 2003.
Covey S. *The Seven Habits of Highly Effective People.* London: Simon and Schuster UK Ltd; 1999.
Dilts RB. *Beliefs: pathways to health and wellbeing.* Portland, OR: Metamorphous Press; 1990.
Dilts RB. *From Coach to Awakener.* Capitola, CA: Meta Publications; 2003.

Evans C. *Time Management for Dummies.* Chichester: John Wiley and Sons Ltd; 2008.

Forster M. *Do It Tomorrow.* London: Hodder & Stoughton; 2006.

Hay LH. *You Can Heal Your Life.* London: Eden Grove Editions; 1987.

Katie B. *Loving What Is.* London: Rider; 2002.

Maslow A. *Towards a Psychology of Being* (3e). Canada: John Wiley & Sons; 1999.

Morgenstern J. *Time Management from the Inside Out.* New York: Henry Holt and Company; 2000.

Neil M. *You Can Have What You Want.* London: Hay House UK Ltd; 2006.

Schechter H. *Let Go of Clutter.* New York: McGraw-Hill; 2001.

Shea M. *The Freedom Years.* Chichester: Capstone Publishing Ltd; 2006.

The Open University: www.open.ac.uk
University of the Third Age: www.u3a.org.uk
Open College of the Arts: www.oca-uk.com
Everyday Health: www.everydayhealth.com
Find out how old you really are: www.realage.com

# CHAPTER 15

# Medicine: a job for life?

Becoming a doctor seemed to be my destiny. As part of a medical family with father, cousins and uncles who were all doctors, following in their footsteps was an inevitable choice, and appeared to be the only possible career option. I did well at school, was interested in people and loved solving puzzles.

Even as a small child I used to play 'hospitals' with my dolls – the game being enhanced with temperature charts my father brought home for me. Mealtimes were interspersed with anatomy lessons as we dissected kippers and chicken legs. All of that combined with a liking for science subjects meant that there was little in the way of discussion of career options, and I followed along the traditional path to a medical future. At that time, in the 1960s, there was a quota for female medical students and for those from overseas. The latter were welcomed more than the former because they were charged high fees, from which the medical school benefited. On the other hand, it was believed at that time that female doctors would not be able to give back as much because they would have children and then want to work part-time. However, it was assumed that male doctors would always want to work full-time.

I enjoyed my time at medical school, apart from the added burden of being 'the professor's daughter' and, as such, having expectations put upon me which I was unable to fulfil, made worse by my father insisting that the local medical school was far superior to others, and that I should apply there. This was compounded by the fact that at that time students could apply for grants which were awarded in relation to parental income. I was only entitled to £50 a year as an award for gaining three A levels at high grades, so as a result was dependent on my parents financially.

However, I survived the years at medical school, living at home initially and then moving into Medical School House – a row of old houses due for demolition, and in the mean time accommodating medical students – during my obstetrics attachment and stayed there until the end of my clinical years.

My determination to leave my home town was very strong, though my father wondered whether I had forgotten to submit an application for local house jobs, and was horrified when I told him I was applying elsewhere, because he believed that my career prospects would be ruined.

However, I wasn't too bothered by these comments, and instead went ahead, read the *BMJ* job adverts, applied and was appointed as surgical house officer in Paddington Green Children's Hospital.

On Friday 1 August 1967 I started my pre-registration surgical house job. Although the hospital was part of the St Mary's Hospital Group, it had only 50 beds in two wards (one surgical and one medical) and a small casualty department.

On the walls of the wards and entrance hall there were Victorian tiled pictures which reminded parents how important it was to keep a window open at night and to bath their child once a week.

I was very keen to start work as a newly qualified doctor, although I felt as if I knew nothing. The first three hours were fine. However, at mid-day everyone went home for the weekend, leaving me the sole doctor in the hospital. I said goodbye to the one other house officer, the registrars, the radiographer, the laboratory technicians and the pharmacist, and was left alone with 50 beds with ill children. Thank goodness for the nurses and the Sister, who knew everything there was to know!

I was on call for not only surgical but also medical paediatric admissions. The registrar was miles away at the end of the phone, reluctant to come in to help me because it was the weekend, and before he would come in I had to take blood, look at it under a microscope (I can't remember if this was to count red or white cells – probably both), examine urine for white cells while seeing kids brought into the casualty department with non-urgent problems which should have gone to their GP. I had (under instruction of the Sister) to take throat swabs, plate these, go to the pharmacy to find the required antibiotics, or arrange for a radiologist to come in if indicated. It was a nightmare. I still feel stressed thinking about it now. What luxury today's junior doctors now enjoy with so many automated procedures!

I had only come across sickle-cell crisis in theory as a medical student, but that was the diagnosis the GP suggested for the first medical emergency I had to deal with that day. I rang the registrar in a panic, and he seemed quite reluctant to come and help me because I hadn't yet measured the child's haemoglobin.

I eventually got used to the daily stresses of the job, and was for ever grateful for the guidance of Sister to set me on the right track.

Next I had a medical house job, followed by obstetrics and gynaecology at St Mary Abbot's Hospital, and by then I was suffering from chronic sleep deprivation, an almost non-existent social life, living in hospital accommodation and eating hospital food every day. I will never forget the sight of a mound of fried eggs floating in a sea of oil on a large stainless steel platter in the doctors' dining room.

I enjoyed gynaecology but not the lack of sleep, so I decided to find some part-time work. As was common at that time, there was no career guidance available, so the only option available for a female doctor who was about to be married and did not want to work full-time was a combination of school and infant welfare clinics, general practice surgeries and family planning.

Other jobs followed, as by then I had a husband and young children and where we lived was very much dictated by the demands of my husband's surgical training. I found suitable work in family planning and general practice, and juggled all of this with kids, general practice surgeries and visits. Moving several times and having to find work which fitted in with family commitments was very challenging.

When my youngest daughter started nursery school I joined the scheme for 'doctors with domestic commitments' who wanted to train for a specialty, and became a registrar in genito-urinary medicine. I particularly liked the 'learning about relationships' part of the job (this was pre-HIV, so the textbook was quite small), and I enjoyed the work very much. However, with the advent of HIV and AIDS the requirements to progress towards consultant status were more than I wanted to take on board at that stage, as I wanted to be able to spend time with my children, too.

Then I moved on to community health clinics as Senior Clinical Medical Officer doing what would now be called 'medical gynaecology', including working with prostitutes, and doing well woman and menopause clinics. I was interested in counselling and achieved a Masters degree in psychodynamic counselling. It was about this time that I attended a workshop based on Louise Hay's book *You Can Heal Your Life*, realised that I very much enjoyed positive psychology and personal development, and also discovered coaching both for myself and as a way to help others.


## RETIREMENT

From doctor to a life after Medicine was a metamorphosis that I experienced in 1997 when I decided to leave Medicine. Of course I was still 'me', but no longer had the label 'doctor', which for 30 years had been very much part of who I was.

The first thing people tend to ask when they first meet you is '*And what do you do?*' There was some status attached to the answer '*I'm a doctor.*' So when I bade Medicine goodbye, I had to find out who I was, and how to define myself without the label.

It has taken me several years to do this, and even longer for my friends to stop introducing me as a doctor. Even now, more than a few years on, if I'm becoming frustrated by an unhelpful pharmacist or outpatient appointment clerk, I tell them 'I'm a doctor' to get the response I want. The way the medical identity sticks is rather like the phantom limb phenomenon after an arm or a leg has been amputated, when the person continues to feel sensations in it.

However, becoming involved with other things has helped me to move away from Medicine into a new identity as a life coach. I have been able to talk to people, listen to their challenges and enable them to find solutions. I have used my medical and life experiences and have developed a niche of coaching doctors.

When I think back to the challenges of retiring from Medicine and forward to retiring from life coaching, I realise that there are various stages of retirement. There is the expectation before the event itself – usually several years of thinking and planning before the actual day arrives. Then, if you are employed, from one day to the next you stop going to work and lose your regular daily routine. It can be quite a shock, and you may react in one of two ways. Either you may do very little at first, enjoying having time to relax, re-charge and plan, or you may leap into hyperactivity and become involved in numerous activities or a lot of travelling.

After a while you may find a middle way. Having regained energy and momentum, you may start to do more or, if you were overactive, you may begin to relax and take life easier. This stage may last for many years unless you are affected by physical or mental infirmity. If this happens you move into the final stages of life by becoming more dependent.

## NOW

As a life coach I help doctors and others to make the changes that they want in their lives and, for anyone preparing for retirement, I facilitate discussion about what has been missing during their working years and what they dream of doing when they retire. It is not my agenda, but theirs. I do not tell someone that what they dream of is possible or impossible. I ask challenging questions so that they can discover for themselves their own way forward.

What I have learned is that life is an ongoing process of change with similar solutions along the way, both for myself and for my clients, whether working in Medicine, considering leaving Medicine before being due to retire, approaching regular retirement age or already retired.

## THE REST OF YOUR LIFE

Beyond having your pension sorted and your will written, what about the rest of your life? How can you prepare emotionally for the changes that are brought about by the life transition called retirement? You can start by deciding what you want for your retirement, and what unfulfilled dreams you now have the opportunity to achieve. Then you can plan the way to move towards those goals by effectively managing your time each day. This means that you have plenty of time for rest and relaxation, but also remain focused on what you want to achieve and so move towards it bit by bit each day. Finally, whatever you decide, you must take action. However wonderful your dreams, nothing will happen unless you are pro-active and take the actions required to achieve them. I could summarise these as follows:

➤ Decide what you want, so that you can work out how to accomplish your goals.
➤ Manage your time, so that you move towards what you want.
➤ Take action, so that you change.

## ADJUSTING TO A NEW IDENTITY

As you may be, I too am going through the process of adjustment, thinking about retirement once more, but not yet quite ready to let go of my current identity. Because I am self-employed, I do not need to stop suddenly. This time it is a gradual process, and meanwhile I am coaching and writing, enabling others to think about and prepare for the lifestyle changes they will go through when they retire.

You have already come to terms with not being the same as before, and being willing to find out who you are becoming. You will notice changes in what is important to you, and what you want to learn and do each day. Your focus may move away from success at work and more towards family and friends and community and looking after yourself than before.

While working, you may always have had too much to do and believed that there was nothing you could do about this. Ways you could have improved things then are even more important when you leave Medicine, because it is easy to spend too much time either doing very little or not doing what you want to do for yourself. Here are some mistakes people make when they retire:

➤ *Agreeing to do whatever you are asked to do.* 'No' is a small word that has a powerful effect. Try it when you are asked to do something. Set your own boundaries and keep to them.

➤ *Not using time productively.* If you regularly spend all day doing very little, plan what you are going to do at the start of each day.

➤ *Doing everything yourself.* You are probably doing several things that you could easily delegate to someone else. Maybe you think it is quicker just to do them yourself, but you may want to pay for some help or do a swap with friends.

➤ *Wasting too much time.* Notice your activities as you go through your day. If you fritter away a lot of time doing unimportant things – for example, watching too much television – spend some of this time doing some of the other tasks that you want to do.

➤ *Not having several different interests.* When you were working you may have been too busy to have any hobbies. You may have used your work as an excuse not to have a social life. In retirement, make your life more balanced. Plan to spend time with your partner, friends and family, or getting involved in community activities.

For myself, I hope that I remain in the active stage of retirement for many more years to come! I am finding time to do things I was too busy to do while working as a doctor. I have written several books and hope to complete more. I enjoy travelling the world and catching up with reading. Visiting grown up children and little grandchildren is my greatest joy and priority.

As for you, do not delay until it is too late to get the best from your retirement and have a life after Medicine.

# CHAPTER 16

# Finally . . .

This book offers you simple suggestions that you can try without further delay to enable you to live the life you truly want after Medicine.

Too many people decide to leave Medicine for whatever reason, and then find that their new life doesn't meet their expectations. They forget their plans and how they wanted to live when they would no longer have the routines of a busy medical job. You, too, may wonder how leaving Medicine will affect you and your perception of life, and hope that you can bring the dreams you had when you decided to leave into your life now.

---

Dr Tree hadn't really made any specific plans for her retirement. In fact Medicine took up so much of her time and energy that she never thought about leaving. Unfortunately, she was suspended while a criticism against her was investigated. Even though she was eventually found to be innocent of the complaint, the investigative process was very exhausting, so she decided not to go back to work but retired instead. However, she became extremely bored and depressed after leaving her job, and all she could think of doing were some GP locums. She found these unsatisfactory, too, and had also become very conscious of everything she did because she feared further litigation. She came to the conclusion that life after Medicine was no better than life in Medicine.

---

Maybe while working as a doctor you kept your personal life on hold until life was more ordered and now, as you are leaving Medicine, you realise that life has moved on relentlessly and you never reached that somewhat mythical time when everything was 'sorted.' You may find it difficult to believe right now, but it's true. There is always transition and change. As some situations improve, other challenges arise. There may never be an ideal time when everything dramatically changes in the way you want. The most important thing, especially now, is to stop putting things off, stop procrastinating, and start to live the life you want now, without further delay.

Perhaps there are practical considerations which mean that you have to keep some things which aren't ideal in your life. Beware of using such excuses as a way to continue dragging your feet. However, now you can begin to introduce what you want into your life and stop doing what you no longer need to do. And when you do that, not only will your life change for the better, but other things will change, too. People around you will change their attitude towards you because when you change you become more focused, more motivated and more able to move towards what you want, and they will change in response to this. A basic principle is that you can only transform yourself, not other people. However, if you become different, other people will alter their behaviour in response, so they will change, too. Remember the systems theory that everything is inter-connected. When you change one thing, other things change as a result. Try it and notice what happens.

You now have the chance to overhaul your life so that you can enjoy life after Medicine. Take the opportunities that are offered, get out there, and follow the suggestions in this book. Be open to new situations and go wherever your spirit leads you. Most of all, become determined that you will have a great life after Medicine.

You know what you have to do and how to do it. All you need now is a large dose of courage to actually take the actions you know you have to take. Like the mother bird waiting for her young to leave the nest and fly, I implore you to jump out and find that you, too, can fly to wherever life after Medicine takes you. I wish you well and lots of fun.

It's never too soon or too late to change your life.

The best is yet to come . . . so get up and make it happen!!

There is life after Medicine. Just like a spreadsheet – change one thing and everything else changes!

For further information, comments or feedback about anything in this book please contact me via the following websites:

www.lifeaftermedicine.co.uk
www.thedoctorscoach.co.uk

# Index